Advance Praise for *Healing Through Yoga*

"Paul Denniston has created a masterwork in grief. He makes the practice of yoga with its wisdom accessible to all experiencing loss. He provides a much-needed beacon to find hope and a healing path forward after the devastation of trauma and grief. *Healing Through Yoga* is truly a helpful companion no matter where you are in the process of loss."

— **Stephen Cope, founder of the Kripalu Institute for Extraordinary Living and bestselling author of** *Yoga and the Quest for the True Self*

"Paul Denniston is brilliant and masterful at getting us to work grief out of our body. He has taken the beloved, ancient practice of yoga and expanded it to include these beautiful heart healing practices. *Healing Through Yoga* is a must-have companion to all whose hearts are heavy with sorrow and grief."

— **Katherine Woodward Thomas,** *New York Times* **bestselling author of** *Conscious Uncoupling* **and** *Calling in "The One"*

"*Healing Through Yoga* is a gentle and insightful guide to help release pain and struggle after even the most devastating losses and to feel and embrace hope. A timely and important book for the world we are living in today."

— **Micah Mortali, author of** *Rewilding*, **director of the Kripalu Schools, and founder of the Kripalu School of Mindful Outdoor Leadership**

"Paul Denniston gently leads us through the cycle of compassionate transformation to break through the struggle and pain of grief and loss. He doesn't ask us to deny or whitewash our feelings but instead guides us to experience them and release them, creating a safe, healing, and fearless path forward."

— **Rhonda Britten, author of** *Fearless Living* **and founder of the Fearless Living Institute**

"*Healing Through Yoga* is an insightful guide to befriending our body and our grief. Through meditations and poses, Paul Denniston helps you to create a space to let go of tension and anxiety and find relaxation and peace within."

— **Joan Borysenko, PhD, author of the** *New York Times* **bestseller** *Minding the Body, Mending the Mind*

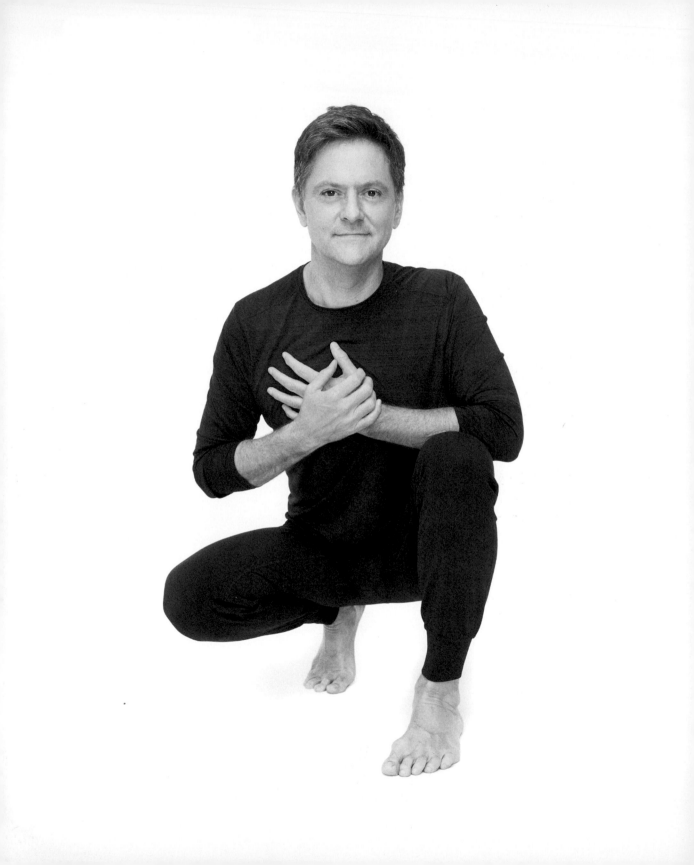

HEALING THROUGH YOGA

YOGA

TRANSFORM LOSS
INTO EMPOWERMENT

PAUL DENNISTON

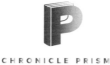

CHRONICLE PRISM

Library of Congress Cataloging-in-Publication Data
Names: Denniston, Paul, author.
Title: Healing through yoga : transform loss into empowerment with more
than 75 yoga poses and meditations / Paul Denniston.
Description: 1st Edition. | San Francisco : Chronicle Prism, 2021. |
Includes index.
Identifiers: LCCN 2021009402 | ISBN 9781797210223 (hardcover) | ISBN 9781797210230 (ebook)
Subjects: LCSH: Grief. | Yoga. | Meditation.
Classification: LCC BF575.G7 .D466 2021 | DDC 155.9/37—dc23
LC record available at https://lccn.loc.gov/2021009402

Manufactured in China.

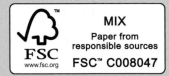

MIX
Paper from
responsible sources
FSC™ C008047
FSC
www.fsc.org

Design by Laura Palese.
Cover photograph by Rob Hyrons/Shutterstock.

10 9 8 7 6 5 4 3 2 1

Chronicle books and gifts are available at special quantity discounts to corporations,
professional associations, literacy programs, and other organizations. For details
and discount information, please contact our premiums department at
corporatesales@chroniclebooks.com or at 1-800-759-0190.

CHRONICLE PRISM

Chronicle Prism is an imprint of Chronicle Books LLC,
680 Second Street, San Francisco, California 94107

www.chronicleprism.com

To my sweet sister,

ELLA,

who I miss every day

Contents

AUTHOR'S NOTE

I wrote this book to present Grief Yoga as a healing tool for loss and to help it become accessible to as many people as possible, so that anyone living with grief, anxiety, or depression may find this practice to be a meaningful tool on a healing journey.

If you have come to this book looking for help, my hope is that this practice offers you a safe space to encourage self-exploration, expression, connection, restoration, and empowerment.

The wonderful people and personal experiences in this book are inspired by my sessions, retreats, workshops, and online discussions with those who have experienced loss. Their names and other identifying information have been changed to preserve their privacy, and some are composites of different individuals. If a real name is used, it is with permission of the individual or is publicly known information.

I deeply appreciate you going on this journey with me toward healing.

FOREWORD

by David Kessler

David Kessler is a grief expert and author of *Finding Meaning: The Sixth Stage of Grief* as well as the coauthor of two books with the legendary Elisabeth Kübler-Ross.

There is no separating the personal from the professional for me when it comes to watching Paul Denniston become the leader in his field of Grief Yoga. I've had a front-row seat to his growth. I often think people come into each other's lives for a reason. When I became a part of Paul's life, I saw that he was using yoga to heal his grief after relationship breakups, but he still had a lot of unresolved grief around death. When someone tells you they avoid funerals, that's usually a clue. I knew it was no accident that the universe brought us together, since my work is all about grief.

I remember inviting Paul to one of my talks about healing after loss. When I was on stage, I looked into the audience and saw that he was becoming more uncomfortable with every word I spoke. I wondered if he would run. Many people do that when they come face-to-face with their discomfort. The next day, Paul's curiosity overcame his fear, and he wanted to know even more about my world. Paul could easily have stepped back, but instead, he stepped forward and committed himself to dig deeper and find healing for himself and eventually for others.

I observed him studying grief and analyzing yoga poses. He came to me with questions as he began applying movement to address loss and healing. Once Paul realized that he could help others navigate and process their loss on the yoga mat, he started to offer small classes in his living room. I was supportive. I didn't know exactly where he was headed, and little did I know that his work and our personal relationship had a promising future.

The word spread about Paul's Grief Yoga classes, but they were limited by the size of the room. I think that local yoga studios were afraid that a class about loss might turn people off, and they were reluctant to bring him in. Then, a few years later, I got a call from Martha Williams, the senior workshop programmer at Kripalu, the well-known, respected, and loved yoga center. She was looking for new kinds of topics to offer the students, and so far, they hadn't done a retreat on grief. She wanted me to lead one.

"I'm glad that you're willing to take on the topic," I told her. Yet I felt a bit inadequate doing a retreat at a yoga center when I wasn't a yoga teacher. I don't even practice yoga regularly. So I told her about the new kind of practice Paul was developing called Grief Yoga. However, since he and I were dating, I said I wasn't in a place to evaluate his work. But I said, "Maybe you could speak with him."

Martha agreed. She found his work interesting and wanted to see it firsthand, but that was difficult because Kripalu is in Massachusetts and we were in Los Angeles. "I'm not the best judge of yoga modalities," I told her, "but when I take Paul's Grief Yoga class, I tear up over old losses."

"That says a lot," she told me. "What if we have him as a part of your retreat, but we won't put him in the brochure. It'll be an add-on bonus, an hour-long class, and I'll watch."

Martha observed Paul's Saturday morning Grief Yoga class and told me she was impressed. She had never seen anything like it. Paul was excited, too, and during an afternoon break that day, we went into the Kripalu bookstore. Looking at the DVDs, Paul said, "I could help even more people who are struggling with a Grief Yoga DVD." In fact, afterward, Paul created several DVDs, and these became the seed for his current online classes, and Paul's hour-long class became a five-day teacher training at Kripalu and led to many other classes in venues around the world.

Paul's work rounds out my approach to grief. I help people deal with their mind and their heart, while Paul's teachings help people process the grief that resides and often gets stuck in their body.

My two teenage sons both loved Paul. About three years after the Kripalu retreat, I got word that my younger son, David, had died. David had just turned twenty-one, and I began drowning in the deepest grief I have ever experienced. I had known deep grief, since my mother died when I was thirteen during a mass shooting across the street. However, the pain of my son's death was soul searing. Paul and I had been together for three years at this point, but I wondered, since the relationship was so new, if he would decide to escape the deep darkness and leave. I knew if I could leave me, I would. But Paul did not. He stuck with me in the epicenter of my horrific loss. A few weeks later, we went to Texas to be with Paul's sister, Ella, who was being hospitalized for stage 4 cancer. At that time, she pulled through, and we went home, only to face the loss of Paul's sweet seventeen-year-old dog, Angel. Paul and I have been together, supporting each other in our journeys, ever since.

I remember Elisabeth Kübler-Ross, my mentor and coauthor, would get so angry when people would try to limit her work to five words—to the five stages of grief she made famous. Or misinterpret them as linear or as five easy steps to grief. Grief is a messy, organic process that unfolds naturally. There is no map, timeline, or straight trajectory. We all do it differently. This book is such a valuable tool for helping us do our own grief work in our own way, at our own pace.

I am proud that this book has found a home at Chronicle Books. So often, we think that grief lives only in our hearts and minds. Paul's work can help us understand that it also lives in our bodies. Our emotions weigh us down and grief gets stuck in our body. Our emotions need motion, and Paul has brought a unique, simple, and powerful way of healing to the world. This book offers an essential tool to help with new and old losses and traumatic experiences that often go unattended. I am honored to have witnessed the birth and growth of such important work.

INTRODUCTION

Growing up in Texas, I wasn't taught how to grieve.

My father was a Baptist minister and my mother was a Christian schoolteacher. They were devoted to God and his word. When they felt sad, they would try to pray it away. So, as a child, I believed sadness wasn't good. Instead, I should just be happy, blessed, and grateful.

This simply wasn't realistic for me. Our human experience on this earth includes all emotions—grief, anger, happiness, peace, harmony, anxiety, depression, joy. This life is filled with all of them. As small children, we don't judge these emotions. We just feel them and let them move through us. When we are sad, we cry deeply and aren't afraid to show it. If we are angry, we have a temper tantrum.

As we become older, we're told that some emotions aren't appropriate. Releasing anger is scary. Feeling sad and crying is a sign of weakness. Judgment of our emotions can isolate us, and then these emotions get stuck inside of us with no way to move through.

My father demonstrated this to me in his belief at the time that it was inappropriate to be angry or to express his anger. He thought that anger should not be felt but instead turned over to God for healing. I wondered if he thought that anger was "ungodly." I watched him hold his anger in, avoid it, and go on with the tasks of his

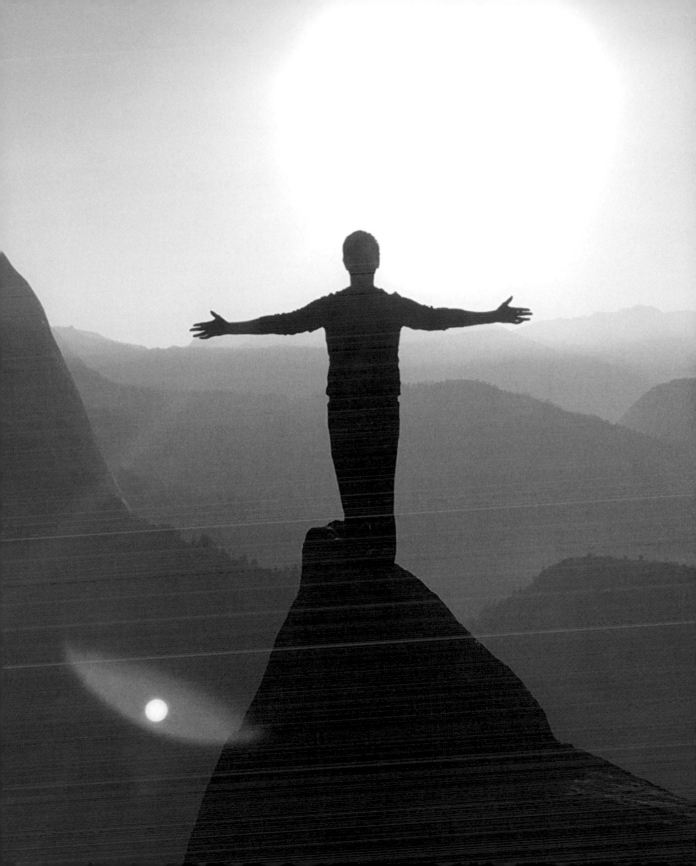

day as it continued to stew inside of him. I remember watching a TV show with my brother that my father thought would be bad for us. He flew into a rage and broke the television. My father, now in his eighties, regrets how he dealt with his anger. I have witnessed his pain and regret; this has been healing for him and for me. I have told him no one is a perfect parent. We all make mistakes. My dad is a very kind, wise man. Yet this is how he was taught to handle anger.

Since I was afraid of intense emotions, if anyone got angry around me, I would look for the door. For many of us, these moments shape not only how we grieve but how we live.

As a child, I suppressed not just anger but all my "negative" feelings. Sadness, anxiety, judgment, fear—I kept them all inside. I isolated myself and was afraid of letting anyone see this part of me, these emotions that I believed were wrong. I didn't know that it was okay to be sad, to be angry—or even to be happy. I compartmentalized so many emotions that I kept myself from joy as well.

Because I didn't know how to deal with these feelings, I used food as an outlet. Fried chicken, chips and salsa, ice cream—these brought me comfort in the moment. As I gained weight, I was ashamed of my body and felt like I needed to hide even more. I became like a turtle in a shell, so much so that even in the hot and humid days of Texas, I wore a jacket that would hide my body. It was my armor to protect me from being seen for who I really was. I wanted to disappear so that no one could see my vulnerability, my wound, my fear, my anger.

Throughout junior high and high school, I was bullied. The judgment that people projected onto me scared me, and so did the hate I felt for them. One day when I was fifteen, Jake, a bully who had picked on me and called me names for years, kept tormenting me in front of everyone at school. I couldn't take it anymore. I pushed him down to the ground and repeatedly kicked him. My anger took over, and I wanted to keep going, but I stopped and looked down at him lying in the grass, hurt and in pain. Was I fighting back at a bully or becoming one? I walked away from that experience believing that my anger was dangerous and needed to be suppressed. I never physically lashed out again. Instead I turned that anger in, beating myself up and telling myself I wasn't enough.

When I was in my twenties, I ran away from any feelings of sadness or grief by becoming active. I put on a happy face and became very busy. When I did experience negative emotions, I avoided anyone or anything that was a "downer" by using drugs or alcohol. I didn't attend my grandfather's funeral, and I avoided my best friend's mother's funeral. I knew her well and disappointed my friend when I wasn't there for him. I avoided sadness, but in reality, I felt *so much* sadness. I carried it with me everywhere.

I felt my body relax and open up. I surrendered to the feelings I was having on my yoga mat.

One day in my late twenties, I attended my first yoga class hoping for a workout and a way to alleviate my anxiety. After ten minutes, I looked around at the other students doing the different poses. Compared to them, I felt fat and awkward. I wanted to appear strong and balanced, but my body was trembling, and my chest felt heavy. I was exhausted and couldn't breathe the way the instructor was guiding me. I wanted to scream. I thought, *Am I about to have an emotional breakdown in front of everybody?* I looked at the door. *Do I make a run for it?* I took a deep breath and thought, *I'll give myself ten more minutes.*

The teacher could see I was struggling and said to me quietly, "You can take a break whenever you need it." Her kindness brought me to my knees. My eyes welled up with tears. I couldn't hold my emotions in anymore and I cried. My mind slowed down and I got more focused. I felt my body relax and open up. I surrendered to the feelings I was having on my yoga mat.

When class was over, I felt peaceful and knew I would keep coming back. In my next few classes, I became curious about where I was experiencing the sensations in my body. I started to tune in to my body and listen to all those feelings from my childhood, and after experiencing the feelings fully, I felt lighter. I felt connected to all my emotions.

For the next ten years, I became a student of yoga. I embraced different types of yoga, and feeling empowered and inspired, I trained to become an instructor myself. My inner child was alive again, and when I received my certification as a yoga instructor, I decided to celebrate by going roller-skating with friends. While I was boogying on the roller rink to Beyoncé, I fell and broke my wrist. A moment of celebration turned to devastation. I had to be in a cast for the next eight weeks, and I wouldn't be able to teach. I didn't even feel like I could be a student.

Everything difficult in my life hit me all at once. My thirty-seven-year-old sister, Ella, told me she had been diagnosed with advanced stage 4 cancer. My sweet old dog, Angel, was sick. I thought her life was winding down. My body was broken, and I felt like my whole life was breaking. I became overwhelmed with sadness. I retreated into my home for months. I used drugs and alcohol to try to numb my pain, and I isolated myself. I overate and became disconnected from the world so no one could see my sadness. I was ashamed of my feelings, and I felt like a failure.

One day, I got sick of it all. I was tired of being stuck and I decided to move forward. For me, that meant going back to yoga, but I was in a cast. I couldn't do the power routine I had done before and I felt frustrated. While everyone around me was moving fast and constantly shifting from pose to pose, I stopped. I slowed my breath and kneeled on my hands and knees. I folded my body into Child's Pose, laying my forehead on the mat with my broken arm by my side, and I began to relax. I allowed myself to have an emotional release where I felt safe from other people's scrutiny. I rested with no regard for what anyone else was doing.

I altered my practice. I stopped doing Power Yoga, and I embraced a gentle and nurturing form of yoga during another teacher training. I grieved the mobility I had temporarily lost. I grieved my sister's loss of health. I grieved my dog's decline. While my arm

One day, I got sick of it all. I was tired of being stuck and I decided to move forward.

healed, I found compassion for my limitations as well as for all the changes in my life. I didn't know it at the time, but this was the beginning of Grief Yoga.

My arm healed, getting stronger than it was before, and what I wanted most was to be of service. Be careful what you wish for. While I was working with the dying in hospice, giving them gentle and compassionate Heart Touch massage, I met David Kessler and we began to date. I really didn't give a second thought to his grief work; I just knew he seemed like a nice guy.

That same month, I was his guest at a large dinner event at the University of Southern California. He was the keynote speaker, and his topic was "How the Death Shapes the Grief." When he began to speak, I felt my hidden grief and pain emerge once again. My breath became shallow. A part of me wanted to run, to make a break for the door. I remembered back to my very first yoga class. I was uncomfortable and anxious, but I decided to stay present instead of running away. I decided to sit in it, listen, breathe, and just be.

As I listened to David speak about guilt and shame, I placed my hand on my belly and focused on my breath. It was difficult, but I knew I was being strong and resilient. I reflected on my sister, Ella, whose body was slowly wasting away with cancer. I didn't know what to do to help her. I placed my hand on my heart and tapped into my sadness. I wasn't avoiding the pain; I was offering myself some kindness. I began studying David's work and became a regular at his grief events.

As I continued to go through more yoga teacher trainings, I took an in-depth look at myself. If I really wanted to help other people, I had to start with me. I was using addictive behavior to numb my pain, and that had to stop. I needed to embody what I was teaching. I made the decision to stop using drugs and alcohol and begin my path to recovery. I got a sponsor, I did the steps, and I allowed myself to feel the struggle and pain instead of numbing myself. I moved with it and through it.

I was also bringing all of my sadness to the yoga mat and finding healing, and I was encouraging others to do the same. One day, David said to me, "You're using yoga for grief." He was right. I decided to create the kind of class that I would want to take—a safe, compassionate container for yoga and movement that honored grief and anger.

What if we used the anger and grief to help us find more purpose, love, and meaning?

My intention with my first Grief Yoga class was to create a ritual that transformed pain and suffering into fuel for healing. What if we moved with grief instead of running away? What if we gave our grief the space to breathe and also honored our resilience and courage? What if we used the anger and grief to help us find more purpose, love, and meaning?

I started teaching Grief Yoga in my living room to friends and students from my current yoga classes. Afterward, we connected over soup and cornbread and talked about our experience.

I expanded my yoga training by studying under yoga masters Gurmukh and Seane Corn. I became a teacher of many branches of yoga, including Hatha Yoga, Vinyasa Flow, Restorative Yoga, Kundalini Yoga, Laughter Yoga, and Let Your Yoga Dance. I learned a great deal from David Kessler, and I wanted to sit in the presence of other experts like Peter Levine, author of *Waking the Tiger*; psychiatrist Bessel van der Kolk, author of *The Body Keeps the Score*; and William Worden, author of *Grief Counseling and Grief Therapy*. I wanted to understand the intersections of grief, trauma, and healing in the body.

I knew that unresolved grief causes a darkness within our life and heart. With Grief Yoga, I was creating a sacred ritual to help turn the light back on. I now teach this class to workshops dealing with all kinds of loss, including breakups, divorce and betrayal, bereavement groups, cancer support centers, addiction groups, groups whose loved ones died by suicide, Alzheimer's support groups, and grieving parents.

I am grateful to travel the world teaching this practice, from the Kripalu Center for Yoga and Health in Massachusetts to the Esalen Institute in Big Sur, California, to workshops and trainings in Australia, Ireland, Canada, Germany, and Mexico. I have seen this work change lives: Susan, a fifty-year-old whose husband left her for another woman, and Mildred, an eighty-five-year-old woman who had never done yoga but was looking for a way to mourn her dead husband. When Mildred did a Dance Prayer (see page 144), she told me she felt like she was dancing with her husband again. I worked with Terrence, an African American man in his thirties who needed to release a deep amount of anger and pain about the racial injustice he had been subjected to all his life, and I guided Janice, a psychologist who needed help processing the death of her daughter due to addiction.

I guided Mandi to help process losing her home to fire, and also Elizabeth who was dealing with the anticipatory grief of watching her mother slowly die from Alzheimer's. I worked with Joshua, who had years of guilt and shame due to his drug and alcohol addiction, and with Isiah, who lost his job and was depressed and didn't know how to move forward. I was of service to Betty, who had been holding on to childhood trauma for decades due to the abuse by her father; to Beth, whose fiancé died in Afghanistan; and to Seth, a teenager who needed to release a deep amount of anger about losing his mother traumatically. I worked with Sandra, a victim of domestic and sexual abuse, who discovered a lump in her breast. She was terrified to have a mammogram because she was afraid to let anyone touch her.

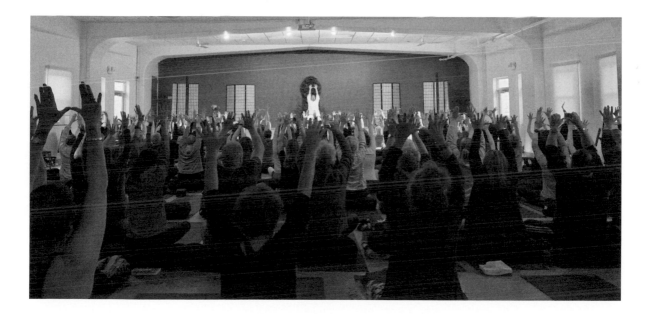

What started out as a way for me to heal the grief in my heart has become a way to help others learn to honor their love by releasing their pain. My mission has always been to use yoga, movement, breath, and sound to release pain and suffering and connect back to love.

Every generation has to deal with collective and personal grief. For our parents and grandparents, it was dealing with World War II, the Vietnam War, and the AIDS crisis. For the current generation, there has been 9/11, hurricanes, the coronavirus pandemic, and the racial injustice that has continued throughout American history. Future generations will have their own losses. Every generation's destiny involves experiencing enormous collective grief, which affects each of us individually.

Yoga provides us with an opportunity to move forward with compassion to heal old wounds.

When the global Covid-19 pandemic changed the world, the loss was insurmountable. All the gatherings and rituals we usually use to process loss had to change, and many were left feeling isolated in their anxiety and grief. When deaths are not witnessed, they complicate grief and disrupt the grieving process. It was shocking and challenging to grasp the depth of it. The number of dead left many feeling shocked, numb, and afraid. Worries about finances and work created deep impacts, both mentally and physically. These psychological and emotional effects will need to be processed for years to come. We all must learn new ways to grieve.

In embracing this book, it's important to take the time to become present and learn to sit with the messiness and chaos of our challenging emotions. Grief Yoga can be a beacon to help you find your way through when you have no idea how to move forward.

EMBRACING YOGA AS A TOOL TO HELP HEAL GRIEF

Yoga can be a saving grace to help deal with grief and loss. We tend to try to distract ourselves from pain through activity, but if we truly want to heal, we need to slow down and be with our feelings. In this way, the *doing* mind softens into the *being* mind, and something powerful can happen on a yoga mat. When we stop and breathe, difficult-to-articulate thoughts and feelings begin to rise to the surface. Yoga provides us with an opportunity to move forward with compassion to heal old wounds.

As we experience our grief, we can get stuck in the past or feel fear and anxiety about the future. But yoga is a pathway to the present, as it asks us to observe the breath and the sensations within the body. When we experience a loss, it can shut us down or crack us wide open. Yoga allows us to befriend our body and our grief, creating a space to let go of tension and anxiety and find relaxation and peace within. As we become present within the body, our wounds will start to surface—wounds of sadness or abandonment can arise for the student to compassionately embrace. The poet Rumi once shared, "The wound is the place where the light enters you."

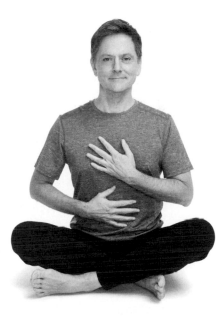

Grief Yoga is an opportunity to release sadness and anger without expectation or judgment. It is a concentrated and gentle opening and stretching of the body with a deep connection to the breath. During some poses and techniques, I'll offer variations to explore what feels right for your body. There is no one "right" way to do this. Observe and notice what is best for you. If this is your first time doing yoga, you'll be comfortable and at ease here. If you've practiced yoga for years, you may find a new perspective within an ancient practice.

THE BRANCHES OF GRIEF YOGA

Grief Yoga is inspired by many different branches and forms of yoga, and it blends them in various ways to help process grief and use it as fuel for transformative healing. This practice is not as much about physical flexibility as it is about emotional liberation. It is a sacred space to express any struggle, and it is a form of surrender, a way to let go of pain and reconnect to love and the gift of life. We use movement, breath, and sound; moving meditations that open the heart; laughter exercises that tap into joy; and Dance Prayers that connect to the soul. You do not need to know about these other types of yoga to do Grief Yoga, but here are descriptions of several important ones (since people often ask).

Hatha Yoga

Hatha Yoga focuses on physical postures to help students stretch, extend, and relax. It helps create balance and grace as we straighten the spine and open the heart. These postures help to improve flexibility and strength, relieving tight shoulders and neck tension. The practice eases back pain and improves breathing disorders and heart conditions. It increases body awareness about the places where stress gets stuck and helps to relieve muscle strain. Hatha Yoga sharpens the mind, empowers the body, and frees the spirit.

Vinyasa Yoga

Vinyasa Yoga is a sequence of postures that stretch and flow, using synchronized breath. You move in a smooth way that flows together like a dance. Focus on the breath is important as you move from one pose to the next on an inhale or an exhale. This meditation of movement and breath helps students find strength and grace.

Kundalini Yoga

Kundalini Yoga is an uplifting blend of spiritual and physical practices that help build vitality and increase consciousness. This transformative practice uses breathwork, meditations, chanting mantras, and kriyas to awaken and connect to our intuition. Kriyas are a specific set of exercises that generate energy to deliver you to a greater sense of awareness as you awaken to your higher self. This powerful practice helps to strengthen your nervous system, balance your glandular system, purify the body, calm the mind, and connect to the fullness of who you are.

Let Your Yoga Dance

This sacred, tribal experience blends yoga, movement, and chakra fusion. You use breath and movement in the seven energy centers of the spine to create liberation, empowerment, and joy. This magical yoga dance helps us surrender the waves of sorrow as we shake off and move through sadness or anxiety. Dancing has immense healing powers to inspire and energize us to embrace self-expression and celebrate life and love.

Laughter Yoga

Laughter can be a medicine to help deepen the breath and allow the flow of emotions to move through. The class follows a mind-body approach to laughter that doesn't focus on jokes or humor, but rather on exercises to strengthen the immune system, bringing more oxygen into the body and brain to help us connect to a childlike playfulness. These laughter exercises mirror daily life and offer us incredible health benefits. Through connection to the breath and exercises, these classes can help shift suffering to create positive feelings.

Restorative Yoga

Restorative Yoga, also known as Yin Yoga, is a series of nurturing postures that allow a gentle approach to stretch and calm the body as you quiet the mind. This practice can be deeply healing for those dealing with trauma, as it allows the body to ease into a pose and remain there for a period of time. Bolsters, blankets, and blocks help you to experience the benefits of a pose without having to exert effort. It can help you find a place of safety and recovery.

THE CYCLE OF COMPASSIONATE TRANSFORMATION

Change is inevitable in life. When experiencing loss, it's normal to experience sorrow, distress, and yearning for things to be different or to be the way they were. We have a strong desire to alleviate heartbreak and struggle. Grief Yoga moves in a cycle of compassionate transformation. It's an awareness that life includes suffering, and it's normal to feel stuck in the midst of the pain. We can choose how to respond to it. We can accept and surrender to what is. Or we can also learn how to expand with it. This is an invitation to be, move, and adapt to the unwanted new normal.

As you move through this cycle of compassionate transformation, I invite you to take this journey at your own rhythm and pace. Perhaps you will need more time to be with a specific step of the cycle. Be gentle with yourself and honor what you need. If you're feeling physical pain, pull back and rest. If you're feeling emotional struggle, I invite you to move forward with curiosity. What can you release using movement, breath, and sound?

Remember, we are slowly transforming every day. Within a transformation, we are undergoing a change in form, condition, structure, or character. We are literally converting from one form of energy to another. This is an opportunity to accept sorrow and to change into something new.

Within this change, perhaps you can identify your distress and find powerful ways to express and release pain. You have an opportunity to sing a different tune. One that demonstrates mercy and tenderness of the heart. One that expresses goodwill toward yourself and others. One in which you recognize that life is changing and you can be open to what today has to offer.

This is an invitation to be, move, and adapt to the unwanted new normal.

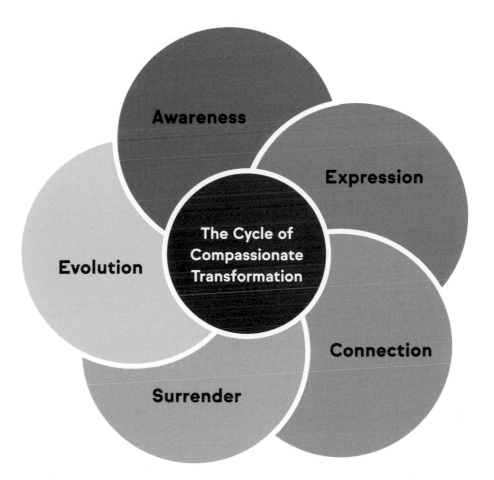

Within this cycle of compassionate transformation, you can alleviate the suffering to guide you toward more grace and kindness. As we move through the changes in our physical, emotional, and mental being, we have an opportunity to mold and reconstruct our lives. This is the cycle we will explore and travel.

This book is organized into five locations along that cycle:

Awareness

This is learning to listen within and find union of mind and body through warm-up exercises and techniques to hear your intuition underneath. So often when we are consumed by grief, we lose our sense of self and our intuition, but that intuition is what will lead us through. We tap into our intuition and emotions just by becoming aware of them again. As we do this, we warm up the spine with breath and movement to become aware of where grief and its accompanying emotions live in the body.

Expression

This is an act of releasing challenging emotions and allowing them to move through you in an intense and powerful practice. Once you've allowed yourself to recognize that you have these emotions, it doesn't help to keep them bottled up inside. Expression asks you to be vulnerable and honest and to expand those emotions beyond your body with courage. This is a way of processing and releasing fear, heartbreak, anger, shame, and guilt. We find powerful ways to move through pain using movement, breath, and sound. Once expression happens, it's time to find healing.

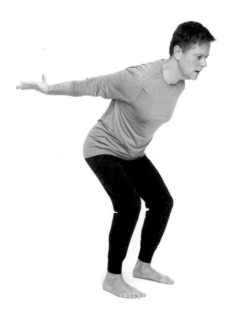

Connection

We are often in a place of struggle and suffering because we're desperately seeking connection and not finding it. After a loss, we often feel isolated and disconnected from those around us. Once you express the struggle, you can shift your pattern and allow a different flow. You may become more open to those emotions you thought you might never feel again, like liberation—even joy. Connection is a process that begins to heal what has been expressed through flowing meditations of grace, forgiveness, love—even gratitude.

Surrender

Many of us are afraid of surrender, but there's something incredibly relieving about it. In fact, it brings us to a place of strength because we become connected to something greater than ourselves. It is a release. A letting go of the pain, not the person. Using restorative postures, you let go of the struggle—but you do not let go of your love. Surrender means that you simply stop clutching at your grief to keep your loved one close. Instead, you keep that closeness by connecting to love.

Evolution

It's possible to move with your grief to discover what might be on the other side: a place of grieving that is empowered, that is strong and alive. Grief is something we all experience, but it is not *who we are*. We are always learning, growing, and evolving. These postures, movements, and breathing techniques help us connect to more courage and resilience as we move forward. We will always have our grief. It is a part of us. And yet there is a reason why we are still here, and it is our ability to connect with others and our own self. Can you be open to the mystery and keep finding meaning in this life?

It's possible to move with your grief to discover what might be on the other side: a place of grieving that is empowered, that is strong and alive.

In reality, you will move through this cycle of compassionate transformation again and again, as you gain more awareness, which leads to new expression, deeper connection, and new growth moving forward. Each step includes a series of specific postures, flowing exercises, and meditations that are specifically designed to move you through that particular step, so that you understand not only what to do but why you are doing it and how it will help. At the end, I offer sample sequences that will guide you through the particular struggle you're experiencing.

Beginning the Journey

Grief is a nurturing caretaker that helps mend a broken heart. It opens the wound and creates space for sadness and longing to breathe. When loss occurs, we long for things to be the way they were. But when we accept the change little by little and sit with the loss, we can connect to a wholeness and resiliency within that can allow us to keep loving.

As you tune in to where your grief lives within, hold that space with loving tenderness. Take care of yourself. Sit with yourself in your sadness. Tell yourself: *When I am lonely and sad and longing for the past, I will nurture my heart and connect to that beautiful vulnerability within.*

The intention and purpose of sadness is to help us see that life is always changing. It can help us recognize what is truly important in this life and keep us moving toward what is fulfilling. The reality is that your grief doesn't get smaller; you must get bigger. You can constantly grow and expand even after great loss. Allow yourself to adapt and change. Flow with whatever heartbreak comes, and move toward the next thing that blossoms in your heart. When one thing dies, another thing grows in its space. Allow your heart to grow.

Grief is a cycle, but one that moves forever forward, and Grief Yoga will help you reach the ultimate goal of returning to a fulfilled, impactful life beyond grief. The thing to remember is that your body never lies. It speaks the truth. When you listen to what your body is trying to tell you, you will see your unresolved sadness and anger—but you will eventually see beyond that. You will see that you are a spirit filled with love.

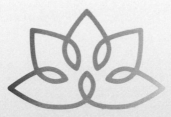

When I am *lonely* and *sad* and longing for the past, I will *nurture* my heart and *connect* to that beautiful *vulnerability* within.

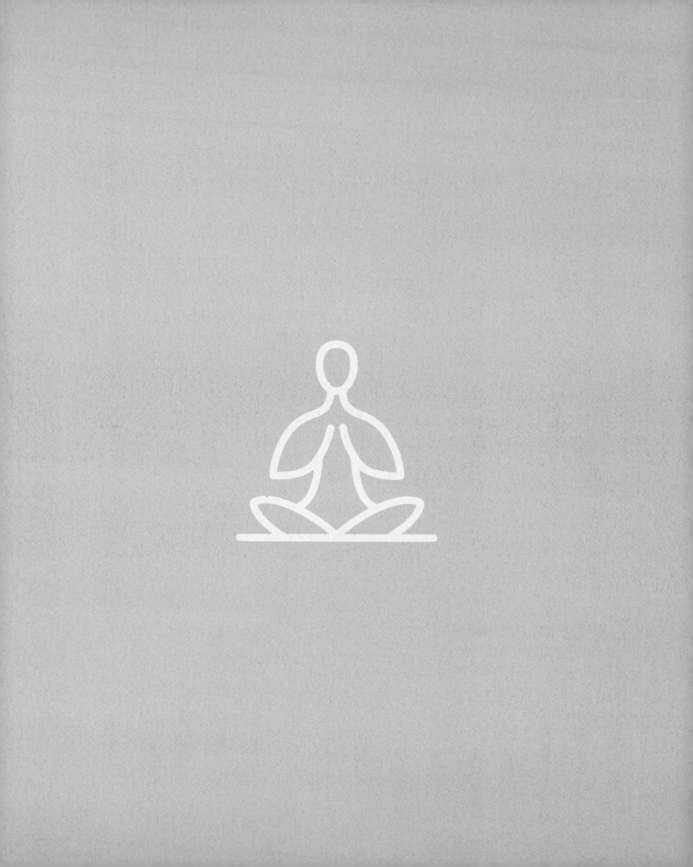

1

Awareness

Neuroscience research shows that the only way
we can change the way we feel is by becoming
aware of our inner experience and learning to
befriend what is going on inside ourselves.

—BESSEL VAN DER KOLK

Awareness helps us to become present, to deepen the breath, to quiet the mind, and to feel safe. When we allow ourselves to feel our feelings, we can identify where the pain and struggle live in the body and encourage it to soften through movement and breath.

We have a tendency to run from our emotions, and this is especially true when we are grieving the loss of a loved one. We move toward distraction, for after all, why would we want to be with this terrible pain? It's so overwhelming. Why would we ever stand still for it?

But there's a paradox in grief: Running from it actually means staying in the pain longer. When we stand still in the pain, we can begin to actually move through it.

Nature understands this. For example, when buffaloes become aware of a storm, they run into it, thus minimizing how long they will be in it. They don't ignore it, run from it, or just hope it will go away, which is what we often do when we want to avoid our storms of emotion. We don't realize that, by doing this, we're maximizing our time in pain. The avoidance of grief will only prolong the pain.

Changing this tendency starts with awareness of our storm. If we don't allow our emotions to come to the surface where we can truly feel them, they get stuck in the body. The body remembers.

Yoga is a moving meditation that allows us to connect to our breath. This focus on the breath helps us to become present and develop awareness of what we're experiencing. When we become aware of our breath, we deepen it.

So often in grief, our breathing becomes very shallow because, when we are experiencing resistance, we constrict our breath. Of course we are resisting our present experience—it is a heartbreaking one, and our life is forever changed. That shallow breath is how we protect ourselves from feeling that heartbreak. But if we can deepen the breath, we can become aware of the feelings underneath that are so hard to be with and process. Yet we must be with them if we are ever to move through our sadness.

DEDICATING YOUR PRACTICE

Leslie came to my class at the urging of a friend, but she didn't really see the point. "I don't know how yoga is going to help when I'm dealing with the death of my husband. This is just going to be too painful," she said.

When we first started working together, Leslie felt a deep resistance to Grief Yoga. She was afraid of moving through her grief. She had been using distraction as a coping mechanism. As long as she kept busy, she didn't have to feel any of her grief. But of course, it wasn't really working. Her grief would bubble up to the surface when she was least prepared to deal with it, and she would have sudden bursts of emotion in seemingly innocuous moments.

As we sat down, I observed how much she was in her head and not in her body. She gazed off as if she wasn't present but, rather, somewhere in the past or future.

I asked her to take a few deep breaths. I could instantly see how shallow her breathing was, how much pain she was in. I asked Leslie to place her hand on the part of her body where she was feeling grief. I told her, "Don't try to fix anything. Just become aware of exactly what it is you're feeling." She placed her hands on her heart, and after a couple of breaths, she stopped and said, "This is too painful."

"That pain is in you all the time," I told her gently. "That pain isn't just here on your yoga mat—you'll take it with you when you leave. Try to sit with it. Let's start by dedicating this practice to the person who died. I'd love for you to say his name."

She looked up and said, "Alex."

The tears started to fall. I wasn't suggesting this to make her feel bad. I wanted to help her feel grounded and to connect what she was doing with the person she was missing with all her heart. This practice, the Hands at Heart Dedication (page 37), is not another "run from" but "a dedication to."

When Leslie felt that the practice had a purpose, it became easier for her to breathe.

She softly said, "I love you, Alex. I miss you." I watched her take this in and release some of her struggle just by breathing.

MOVEMENT

Leslie and I began to warm up the spine. Since she was holding so much tension in her throat, we started with her neck (doing Neck and Shoulder Release, page 40). While she was seated on her mat, I had her do some neck rotations. We carry a great deal of stress, tension, and anxiety in the neck and shoulders as byproducts of our grief. Bringing awareness to this tension allows the breath to come in, open up, and loosen. From there, Leslie began shoulder rotations. She flowed with her breath, moving her stiff shoulders in one direction and then the other. I told her, "Grief lives in our heart, mind, and body. Our heart handles grief naturally, but we can get stuck in our mind as we try to think our way out of the pain." This movement helped her get out of her head and become aware of the sensations within her body.

We carry so much emotion in our joints, our tendons, our muscles—in our very cells. If we don't feel our emotions, they get stuck inside of us. But we can acknowledge them, fully experience them, and then let them go.

When our heart is broken, as Leslie's was, we don't notice how our body constricts. Leslie needed to go slowly because she was feeling so much. She was filled with emotions that she'd been resisting for a long time, and she needed to be gentle and tender with herself.

She and I shifted into a flow I call Torso Twists (page 44), which rinses the body out like a washing machine, letting go of the hurt and resentments that are coming to the surface. Grief is more than simple sadness. We can be angry; we can feel guilty, afraid, and ashamed. These are normal reactions to loss, but because they are painful and confusing, we want to hide or run away from them.

Loss causes us to twist and change in ways that we are not ready for, that we don't want. We tense up to protect ourselves, and so the spine becomes rigid in grief. Grief needs motion. For Leslie, this movement allowed her to loosen at her own pace, gently, so that she could adapt to this new way of being with less struggle.

I asked Leslie to place her hands on her knees and move into Sufi Grind (page 48), a circular movement of the torso, with her sit bones grounded into the earth. When we experience a loss, it feels like our life is caving in. We need to make space and build ourselves up again. These large circles of the torso create that space, and they also awaken the heart.

"It feels good to just move," Leslie said. "I've felt stuck for a while. There are a lot of feelings bottled up inside of me."

I looked at her and said, "Perhaps you've been trying to think your way out of grief with all your distractions."

"I think you're right." She suddenly laughed. "There I go, thinking again!"

In grief, the torso tightens up because of the stress. This is our primitive fight-or-flight response to protect a wounded heart, so we need to open the torso back up and move it around. We are still alive. We need to move through the struggle.

AWARENESS TECHNIQUES AND EXERCISES

As you can see from Leslie's process, if you focus on the body, you quiet the mind. As you deepen your breath, the union of mind and body will help lift the spirit.

Have you ever been caught up in emotional turmoil, like a fight with a friend or loved one, and gone for a walk? We feel called to take that walk because we know intuitively that movement can help us process our feelings. As we walk, we experience and become aware of our emotions and start to move through them.

Yoga is a mixture of movement and stillness. When you practice Grief Yoga, you move your energy. Emotion is energy in motion, and movement allows us to help release the pain and struggle to find our flow.

Stifled emotions weigh us down. The following poses, flows, and moving meditations will help you float, rather than sink. Just move.

We carry so much emotion in our joints, our tendons, our muscles—in our very cells. If we don't feel our emotions, they get stuck inside of us.

Seated Grounded Breath

———

When experiencing grief, we can get stuck in the past or feel fear and anxiety about the future. This grounded breath helps us to become present. As we observe our breath, it will help quiet the mind so that we can become more connected to whatever we're feeling.

1. From a comfortable seated position, close your eyes and become aware of your connection to the earth, to where your body is touching the mat.

2. Check in with yourself by performing a body scan. Do you feel physical or emotional pain? Where? Observe where tension lives in your body. Bring attention to the sensations within.

3. As thoughts arise, observe them and return attention to your breath. You can also put one hand on your belly and one hand on your heart and silently whisper, "Body, breath." This can help you tune in to how you're feeling in this moment.

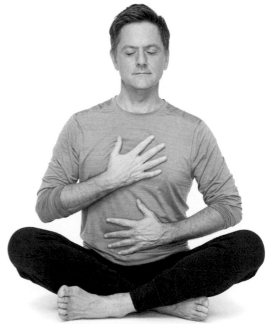

4. Continue for one to three minutes, observing your breath and holding that space with compassion.

Hands at Heart Dedication

———

Dedicating your practice to the person who has died can be deeply powerful. Your heart misses them. Honor your love by reflecting on the person and dedicating your practice to the love you shared.

1. From a comfortable seated position, place both hands on your heart and close your eyes.

2. Tune in to your breath and connect to your heartbeat and to your heartbreak. Envision the loss that weighs heavy on you and hold your heart with care.

3. With your mind's eye, see your loved one who has died, the person you want to see more than anything. Perhaps say their name out loud. Dedicate this practice to them. Dedicate it to the love you feel.

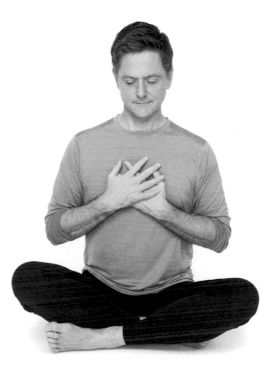

Jaw Release

———

It is difficult to speak about our anxiety, hurt, and pain, but if we don't, we can carry that pain in our bodies. Release tension in your jaw using movement, breath, and sound.

1. From a comfortable seated position, bring your hands in front of you and clasp your palms together.

2. Inhale through your nose, and as you exhale through your mouth, shake your palms together in front of you and release any tension in your jaw. Visualize the tension moving from your jaw down into your chest and out through your hands.

3. Also as you exhale, use vocalizations without words. Play with any type of sound, whether it is quiet or loud, long or staccato, atonal or musical. Release the tension in your jaw as you explore with sound, tone, and the vibration of your voice.

4. Continue this inhale/exhale exercise three more times.

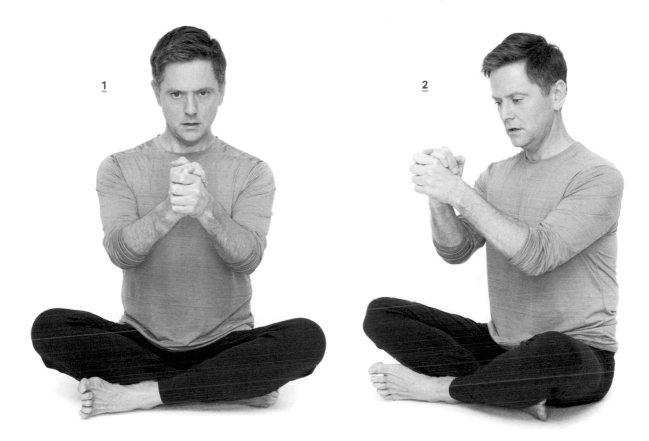

1

2

SOFTEN THE JAW

We often hold tension in our jaw because we have a hard time sharing about our loss. Society doesn't want us to talk about grief. Or others want us to talk, get it out in the first week, and then be done with it and move on. We mistakenly think we need permission to talk and grieve. Sometimes this tightening of the jaw can be unconscious. Many people have told me how they start grinding their teeth at night. We must release grief during the day or it finds us at night.

Neck and Shoulder Release

———

Grief can feel like we are carrying a backpack of guilt, shame, anger, and sadness that our neck and shoulders can't shrug off. We hunch over, feeling defeated by life and loss. We fight the loss rather than fighting to drop it entirely, allowing some breath and movement to help us open up and let some of that weight go.

1.   From a comfortable seated position, bring one ear to the nearest shoulder, then your chin to your chest, then bring the opposite ear to the other shoulder, and repeat, drawing large circles with your head.

2.   As you do, breathe into your neck and shoulders, bringing in fresh oxygen. Keep rotating for a minute, then reverse direction, ear to shoulder, chin to chest, opposite ear to your other shoulder, for the same amount of time.

3.   Find your own pace; go slowly or quickly. Regain a sense of the control you have lost. Allow this to feel good. This motion brings oxygen to the brain.

4.   Once the neck rotations are complete, move into the shoulder release. On an inhale, bring both hands to your heart in tight fists and lift both shoulders to your ears. As you exhale, allow your hands to relax and come back down to the knees as you lower your shoulders. Be aware of any tension that remains and soften it with each repetition.

5.   Continue the shoulder release three more times, then come back to your natural breath.

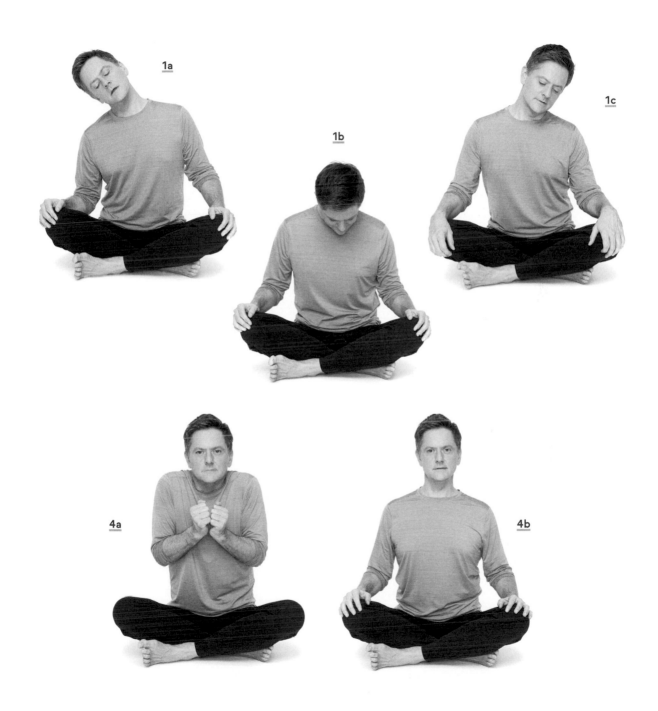

41

Spinal Twist

If you're feeling anxious or overwhelmed, Spinal Twist can help you feel more grounded, stable, and balanced, physically and emotionally. These twists create space between the vertebrae to provide added blood flow to the spine. After this, if you'd like to move and twist the spine further, do Torso Twists (page 44).

1. From a comfortable seated position, place your left hand on your right knee. As you inhale, lengthen your spine upward. As you exhale, twist and gaze over your right shoulder. Continue two to three more times as you gently twist on your exhale.

2. Come back to center and place your right hand on your left knee. As you inhale, lengthen your spine upward, and as you exhale, gently twist your spine and gaze over your left shoulder. Continue two to three more times on this side as you gently twist on your exhale.

3. Repeat by gently going back and forth on both sides, and if you'd like to stay a little longer on one side to go into a deeper twist, please do.

4. Continue at your own pace for one to two minutes. When complete, come back to a neutral seated position with your sit bones balanced and your spine straight. Breathe deeply.

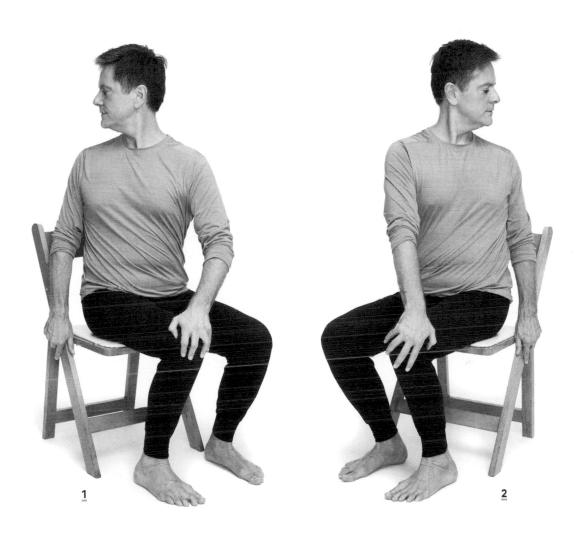

1

2

Torso Twists

———

Imagine grief as weight. Grief weighs down your spine, sometimes literally compressing the vertebrae. To help us move forward and create space for our grief, we have to elongate and move the spine.

1. From a comfortable seated position, place your left hand on your left shoulder and your right hand on your right shoulder. Bring your fingers forward toward your chest, thumbs pointing back, elbows raised at shoulder height.

2. Do Torso Twists from side to side. Inhale and twist left, then exhale and twist right, gently twisting your spine. Repeat the motion without pausing; inhale left, exhale right.

3. As you twist with your breath, rotate from your navel point, and allow your chin to remain in line with your chest. Relax your muscles and move easily as you gently open and twist your torso.

4. Continue at your own pace for one to two minutes.

TWIST AND TURN

During Torso Twists, you may feel some resistance to all of these twists and turns. Your life has taken a turn you didn't ask for, one that left you feeling helpless. But that turn came and more will come. This twist and turn is something you can control. In the past, it may have felt like all you could control was your own tension, your own need to carry this weight. Now, allow yourself some movement.

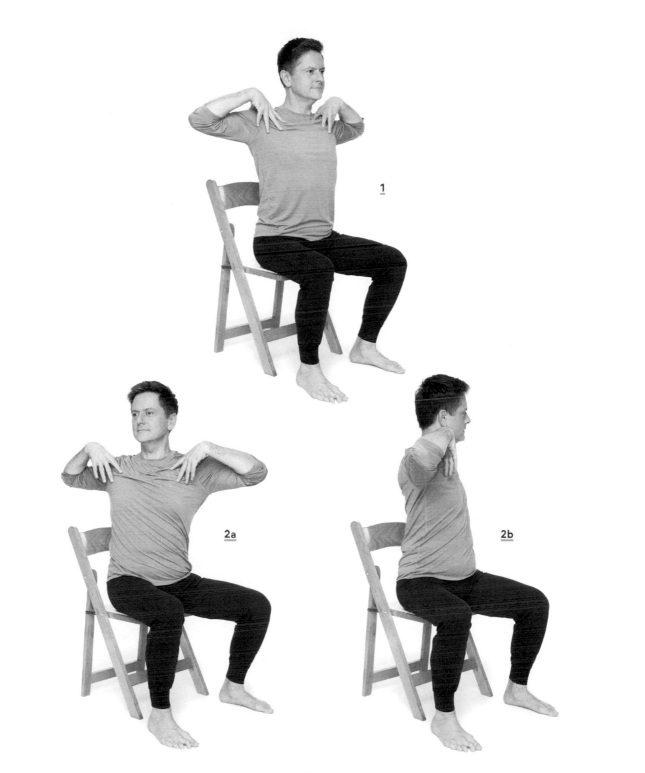

1

2a

2b

45

Side Stretch

___

In grief we all experience yearning. The longing for the person just out of reach in the physical world. Sometimes it helps to embody that yearning. Perhaps you believe your loved one is in heaven or the afterlife. Make your yearning experiential with this stretch. You have been emotionally stretching to be with them; now use your body. Be aware of where you're touching the earth and how your body feels as you breathe.

1. From a comfortable seated or standing position, lift your hands above your head and breathe deeply.

2. Lower one hand down to your side and reach the opposite hand up over your head, stretching to the side with the lowered hand. As you stretch, take a few deep breaths in and out.

3. Straighten and lift both hands up, then lower the other hand to your side and reach the still-raised hand over your head, stretching to the other side. Breathe into that bend.

4. Continue stretching back and forth at your own pace for one to two minutes. Flow with your breath from one side stretch to the other.

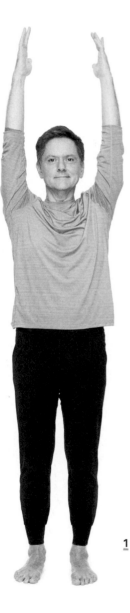

1

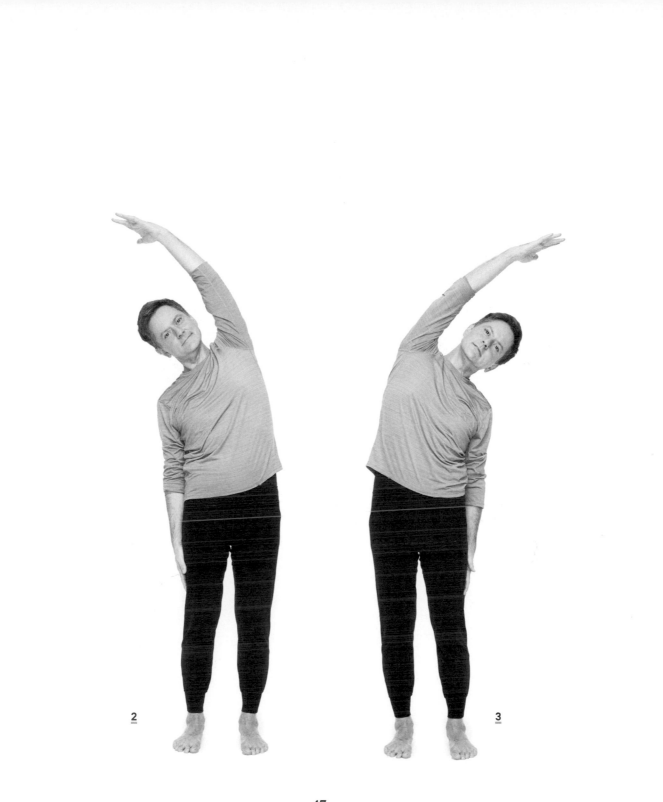

2

3

Sufi Grind

———

Remember that even in deep loss, love still exists. This practice will create movement and space for that love—love that you may not be able to feel right now, but it is there. Strong emotions can come up in this movement, like anxiety and sadness, and that's okay. Just let any emotions be with you as you move.

1. From a comfortable seated position, place your hands on your knees. Moving from your waist, circle your torso in one direction, shifting forward, to the side, back, to the other side, and so on.

2. Continue making large circles as you observe your breath. Connect to your core for support as you gently open and move your spine.

3. After one to two minutes, reverse directions, repeating the same large circles with your torso, at your own pace, for the same amount of time.

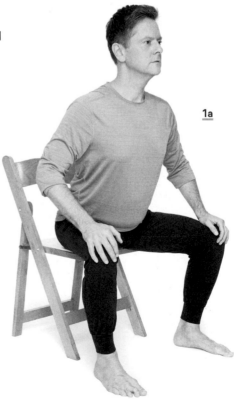

1a

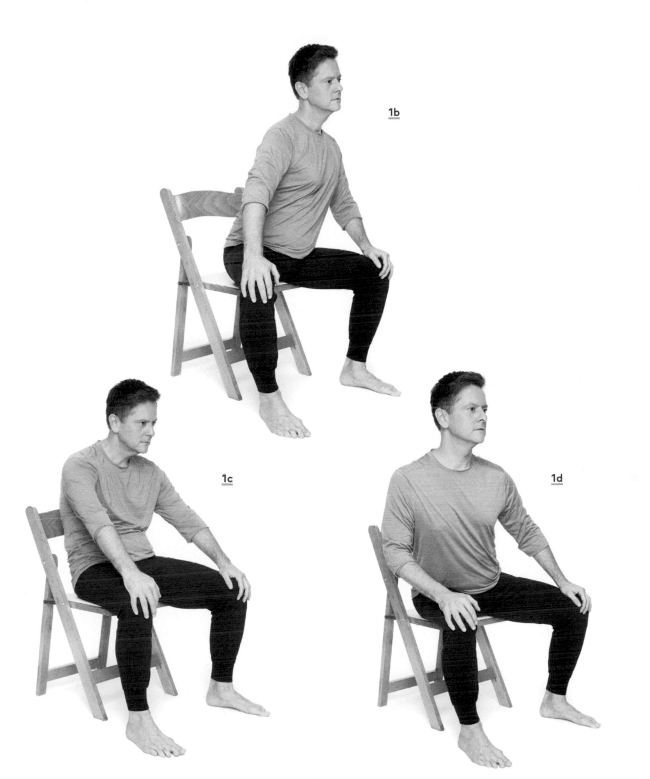

1b

1c

1d

Cat/Cow

———

You can quiet your mind and move through pain by observing and flowing with your breath. Whatever emotion you're experiencing, it's important to let it move through you. This flowing meditation guides you toward more emotional balance as you relax the muscles in your back and strengthen your spine. Many people who practice yoga are familiar with Cat/Cow. The next pose, Swan, builds on these poses to achieve more flow.

1. Assume a tabletop position on your hands and knees. Place your palms directly under your shoulders and your knees beneath your hip bones, keeping your back straight in a flat, neutral position.

2. As you exhale, move into Cat pose by pressing your palms down as you round your spine like an angry cat; draw your shoulder blades away from each other and your chin to your chest.

3. Continue as you flow with your breath: Inhale into Cow pose, with belly down and gaze up, then exhale into Cat pose, spine rounded and chin to chest. Feel the rhythm with your breath as you gently move your spine.

4. Continue at your own pace for one to two minutes.

VARIATION

If kneeling in tabletop position is uncomfortable, sit forward on a chair with your hands at your knees, and move your spine and shoulders in the same way. As you inhale, move into Cow pose by lifting your tailbone and lowering your belly; draw your shoulder blades toward each other and lift your head, gazing up.

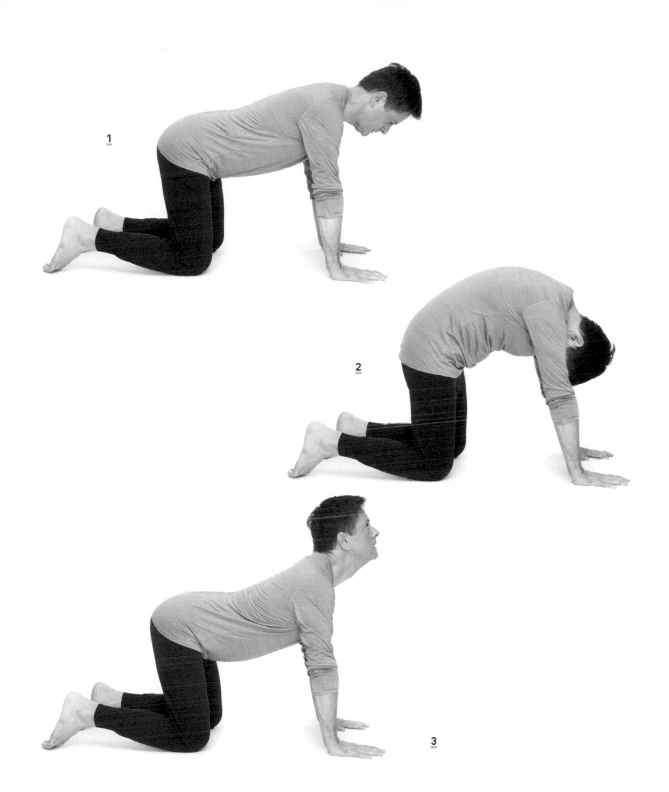

Swan

———

We often think of grief as a storm. As you move through this flowing pose, allow a sense of grace and ease to move like a wave through your body. The turbulence is still there, but you can move your heart smoothly through it, at your own pace, in your own rhythm.

1. Assume a tabletop position on your hands and knees, with your shoulders over your wrists and your back straight. Breathe deeply throughout this flowing meditation.

2. Lower your chest toward the earth, bending your elbows.

3. Extend or lean your head forward and then round your spine up.

4. Bring your chin to your chest and your hips toward your heels.

5. **Continue this flow:** Inhale as you bend your elbows and arch your spine down, then exhale as you round the spine back up and bring your chin to your chest and your hips toward your heels.

6. Continue at your own pace for one to three minutes. When complete, come to stillness in the tabletop position and observe.

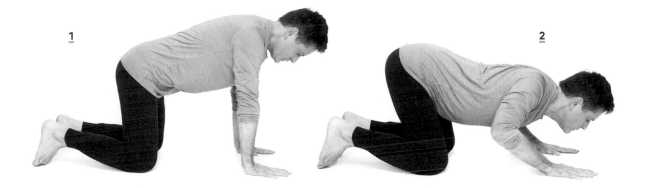

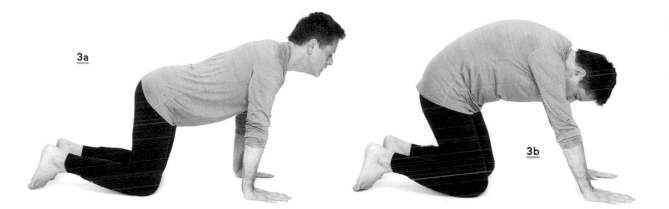

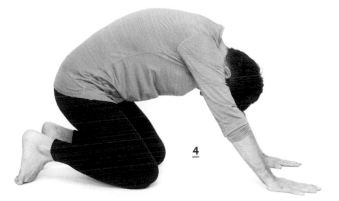

53

Child's Pose

If vulnerable feelings are coming up, allow yourself to feel the support of the earth. This pose represents being cared for and caring for yourself. The head angles downward so the heart can rest and allow blood to rush or settle to the brain. This is a pose to rest, to take care of yourself, and to feel whatever is there.

1. Kneel on the floor, knees spread wide, and sit back on your heels.

2. Fold your upper body forward, guiding your head toward the floor. If your hips lift off your heels for your head to reach the floor, that's okay. Explore what feels right for your body and find safety. Lay your arms comfortably on the floor, either beside you or in front of you.

3. Close your eyes, empty your mind, feel your feelings, and observe your breath. Rest in this position for as long as you want.

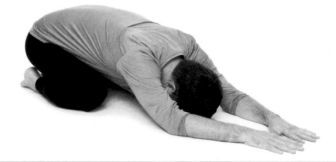

TURN INWARD

This nurturing posture provides a place of protection. Whenever you feel overwhelmed, return to Child's Pose and take a moment for yourself. You can turn inward like a turtle coming into a shell. You can release tears without anyone seeing you.

Bumblebee Hum

———

This breathing practice provides a place to rest and soothe your feelings. It helps you connect to your vibration, so that you can hear only yourself. The vibration sounds like a bee humming in your head. There is something incredibly soothing about vibration—it quiets both the outside world and our own mind.

1. From a comfortable seated position, relax your body and breathe deeply in and out through your nose.

2. Place your thumbs in your ears, blocking any external sound, and lay your four fingers over your eyes, blocking any light.

3. Inhale deeply through both nostrils. As you exhale, make a deep humming sound in the back of your throat. The exhalation and hum are smooth as you connect to your vibration within.

4. Continue breathing and humming in this way for one to three minutes.

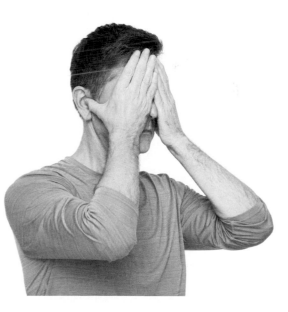

Runner's Lunge

We carry a lot of suppressed emotion within our hips. As we open them up, we can learn what's there. The Runner's Lunge helps us embody our intention to move through grief. This posture prepares our body and mind to get ready to move through the place where we are stuck.

1. Assume a tabletop position on your hands and knees. Bring your right foot forward and place both hands inside your front foot. Allow your back leg to straighten, and either relax it behind you with your knee on the ground or tuck your back toes under and lift your knee off the ground.

2. Breathe into your hips as if they were lungs, and as you exhale, sink deeper into that stretch, allowing the pelvis to relax. Your hands can be under your shoulders for support, or for a deeper stretch, come down onto your forearms. Hold for a minute, then return to a tabletop position.

3. Repeat on the other side. Bring your left foot forward and place both hands inside your front foot. Allow the back leg to relax or tuck your back toes and lift your knee off the ground as you breathe into your hips. Hold for a minute.

4. When complete, come back to the tabletop position or rest in Child's Pose.

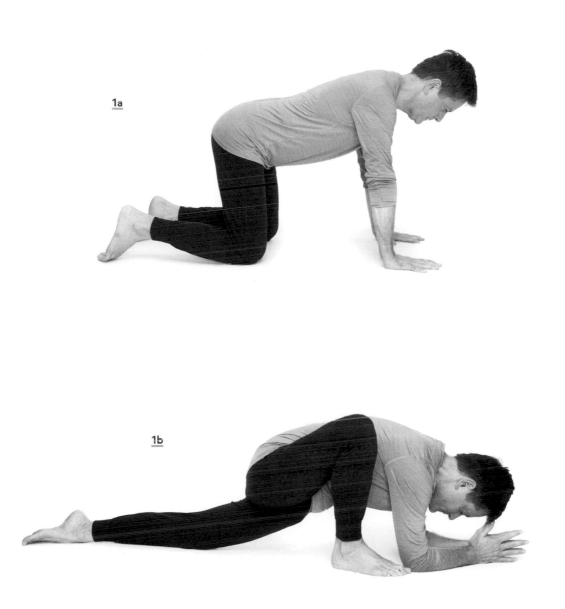

1a

1b

Waterfall

In loss, you're literally bent in half. As you fold your body forward, blood and oxygen run down your spine toward your head, like a waterfall pouring down toward the earth, releasing tension and stress.

1. Stand with your feet parallel and hip-width apart.

2. Bend your knees slightly as you hinge from your hips, folding your upper body forward while breathing into your lower back. Release your arms to the ground and allow your head to be lower than your heart.

3. Shake out and release any tension in your shoulders and neck.

4. Hold for one minute and slowly come back up to a standing position.

FIND STABILITY

When we've experienced a deep loss, it can feel like our life and world have been turned upside down. Your head is drooping toward the earth. But even in that space, you can still feel grounded to the earth and find stability in the soles of your feet and in your breath. Try to connect to that sense of stability, even if it feels gone entirely. It is always there, ready to support you.

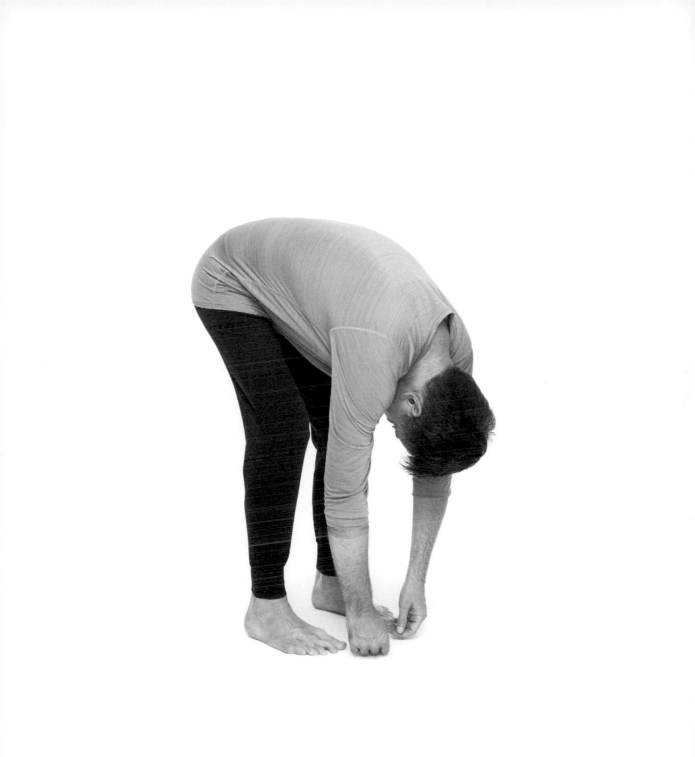

Flowing Breath

This practice moves oxygen and energy up and down the body, with the intention of bringing the burden up and out and inviting the healing down. You can lift up your struggle and raise it over your head like an offering. As you exhale, bring the healing down to the earth. As you do, really feel your feet on your mat, rooting you into the present.

1. Stand with your feet parallel and hip-width apart. Bend your knees slightly with your hands at your sides.

2. Inhale and, with your palms up, raise both arms up and over your head.

3. Exhale and, with your palms down, float both arms down to your sides as you relax your shoulders, keeping your knees slightly bent.

4. Continue at your own pace, without pausing, for two to three minutes. Let your breath flow with the movement as if you were moving through liquid or air.

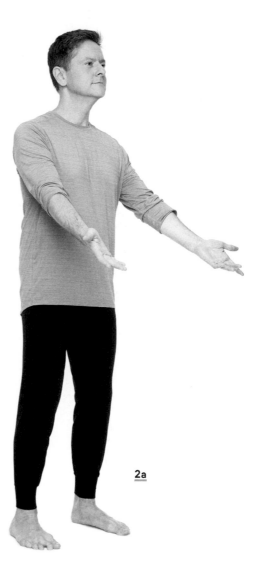

2a

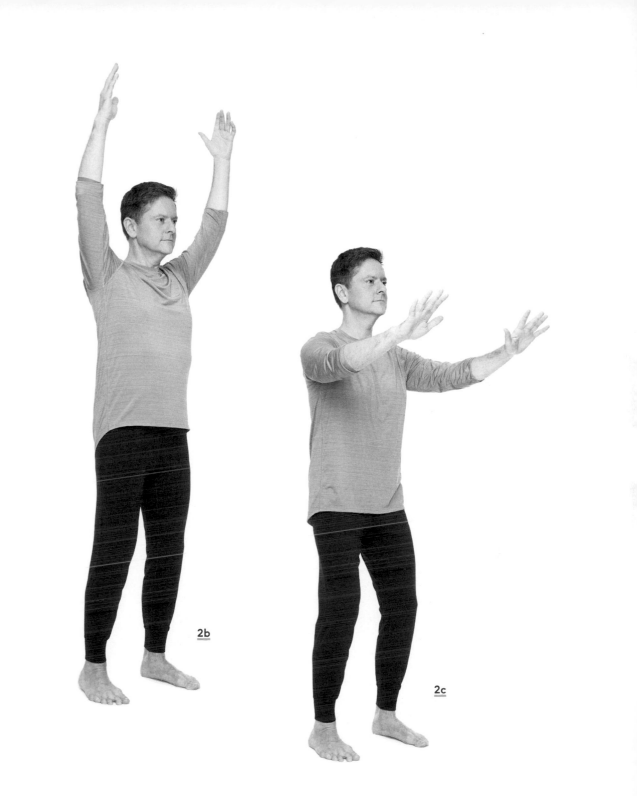

2b

2c

Phoenix

───

As we move through our grief, sometimes we open and expand; other times we contract. The truth is we may need to do both for a while. At times, you may want to turn away from and deny your grief. Denial is the act of moving from reality to distraction. It's okay to get distracted. You can touch the pain and then walk away from it. Use this technique to curl around it, absorbing it.

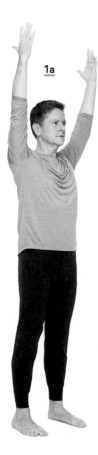

1a

1. From a standing position, inhale as you bring your arms up over your head. As you exhale, continue into a gentle backbend, bending your elbows with your palms up. Feel your heart opening. Hold for a moment, breathe, and open your chest.

2. Inhale and straighten your back, keeping your arms raised. Touch palms, and as you exhale, bring your hands through the heart center and fold your upper body all the way forward, bending at the waist. Breathe deeply and then lift your upper body till it rises halfway; place your hands on your shins and create a flat back by extending your tailbone back and your chest forward. Hold and breathe as you lengthen your spine from your tailbone to the top part of your head.

3. When ready, lower into a squat by bending your knees, lifting your heels, and bringing your forehead to your knees. Curl into a compact little ball. Hold for a couple of deep breaths, then return to a standing position.

4. Continue at your own pace for one to three minutes, repeating the entire sequence. As you move up and down, you are opening your heart, and then retreating and protecting it.

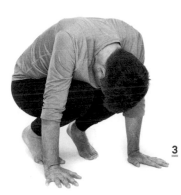

1b

2

3

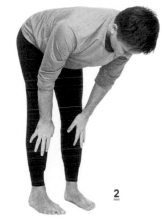

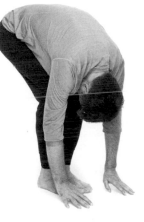

VARIATION

If a squat and curl is uncomfortable on your knees, instead fold forward at the waist, letting your hands drop toward the ground, forehead toward your knees. Breathe deeply.

Moving into Expression

After these moving meditations, you're likely more aware of some intense emotions. This is not a comfortable place to be, but know that Grief Yoga is a safe space. It's important to move these challenging feelings through you—and the way to do this is by expressing them.

In the expression exercises and techniques, we move and breathe in some powerful ways, incorporating sound and tapping into our fire to help release the struggle.

63

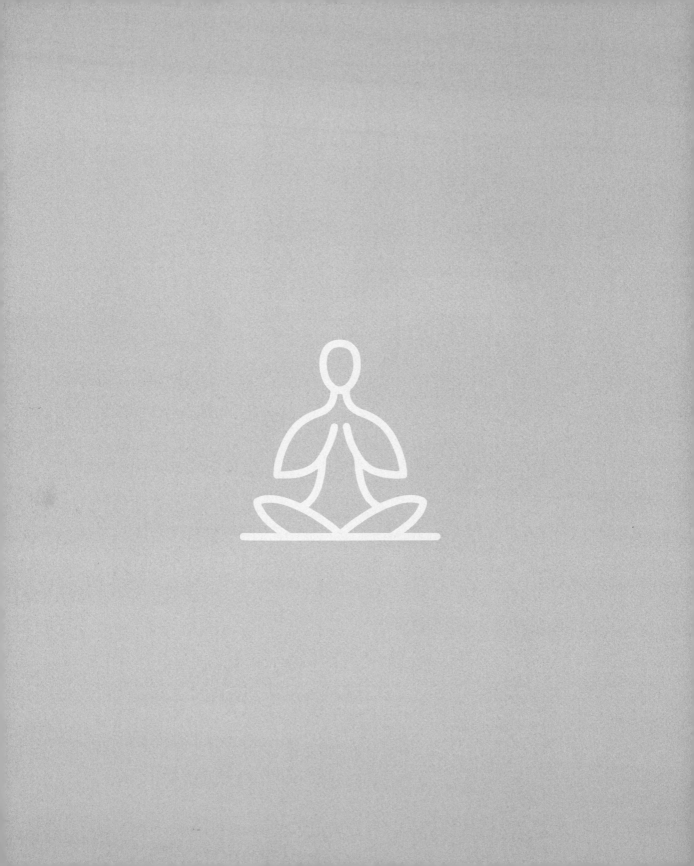

2

Expression

Expression is the opposite of depression.

—EDITH EGER

Expression uses movement, breath, and sound to help release the hurt and struggle. We are tapping into our fire within, and we are using our pain as fuel for healing to help guide us forward.

Many people experiencing grief try to avoid challenging emotions or to push them down. Or sometimes someone tries to express their feelings to friends and family, only to discover that those people are not as safe or open as the person hoped. Others might try to avoid someone's grief by telling them to get over it and move on.

It can be surprising or hurtful when those closest to us, our dear friends and family, just don't get it. We end up covering over our challenging emotions and keeping them bottled up inside. This is self-protection. I know from my own childhood that suppressing feelings can sometimes be necessary, and that running from grief and anger can last decades. I was taught not to express challenging emotions or grief, and I never want to make anyone feel wrong for pushing feelings down.

You may be in survivor mode, and grief might feel like a luxury you can't afford at this particular time. However, when you are stronger and have built a safer foundation, the grief will appear, since it still needs to be expressed. This work provides a safe place to express all that lives inside.

THE IMPORTANCE OF EXPRESSION

To express yourself is to share a part of yourself, and that takes courage, since sometimes other people won't like it and will judge your expression. Many of us were raised to be people pleasers. We all suffer from the fear of being judged. We judge others. Others judge us. We judge ourselves. We judge our feelings.

Judgment isn't always negative. Sometimes it's a useful tool to help us discern the difference between good and bad. To some extent, in different ways, everyone is raised to distinguish good from bad, since this is an early tool to help us navigate the world. As adults, we can use our judgment to identify what needs work and how to make things better. Judgments help us explore our choices and see if anything needs changing.

Many times, however, judgments are also surprising and painful. That's the reality of the world in which we live. If we accept the truth of living in a world of judgment, then we can decide how to maneuver within it. How many people go from one disappointment to another within their friends and family, feeling constantly hurt by judgments? However, what if we understood humans as judgment machines? That way, we would expect judgment, rather than be constantly disappointed by it. We would live in freedom. We don't need to fear being judged once we acknowledge that we will always be judged. By accepting the world as it is and learning how to handle its judgments, we will improve our ability to freely express who we are and how we feel, including our deepest emotions—that is, our fears, heartbreak, anger, shame, and guilt.

Judgments don't just come from others. We also judge ourselves. However we handle our difficult emotions, our inner critic often judges us as doing it wrong. We express too much or not enough, or to the wrong person or in the wrong way. Our inner critic builds a case against us out of fear of being hurt. I like the saying that the word *fear* is really an acronym that stands for "false evidence appearing real." We fear what *might* happen, without knowing what *will* happen, and courage arises when we recognize our fears, express our fears, and move forward anyway. Remember, courage isn't the absence of fear, but going on in spite of it.

Many of the people I work with are afraid of dropping into grief because they feel like they'll never come out of it. They say things like, "If I go there, I'll never be able to recover. I'll be stuck in the depths of sadness." But if grief doesn't get expressed, it stays stuck inside. If someone is already *in* those depths, expressing their emotions allows them to move through so that they can move forward.

> # If we accept the truth of living in a world of judgment, then we can decide how to maneuver within it.

SUPPRESSED EXPRESSION

Wanda, a married woman in her thirties, is a student of mine. For many years, she was dealing with a lot of anticipatory grief (grief before a loved one dies) as she watched her mother, who lived in a nursing home across the country, slowly deteriorate in mind and body.

During the coronavirus pandemic, Wanda's mother got sick from Covid-19. Wanda couldn't fly to be with her, and she could only speak to her through Face-Time. Wanda felt overwhelmed with trying to make sure her mom was okay and with trying to hold it together for her family. When her mother died two weeks after being diagnosed, Wanda had to arrange a funeral on Zoom.

Afterward, Wanda and I connected on a Zoom Grief Yoga class. Her shoulders caved in as if the weight of the world was weighing her down. I saw the pain in her eyes as she gripped her fists tightly, trying to keep in all her emotion.

"You look angry," I said, "which is totally understandable."

Wanda gave a frustrated laugh. "Mom taught me it wasn't appropriate for girls to be angry. It's hard for me to express anger. I never felt like I could."

"I see how much pain you're in. I'm not here to fix you, but I can offer some tools to help you move some of the pain through. Would that be okay?" I asked her.

She nodded. I invited her to deepen her breath. As we went through several awareness techniques to warm up her body and spine, the rigidity in her body began to soften and flow.

"Stand up, Wanda," I said.

She snapped back with an intensity I had not seen. "Don't tell me what to do!"

"Yes, that's it, use that anger. I want to help you move the anger through using what I call the Woodchopper. I *invite* you to stand up."

She stood, and then I softly guided her through the Woodchopper (see page 80). This technique mimics chopping a piece of wood, so that you imagine holding an ax and bringing your arms down while yelling "HA!" as loud as you can.

As Wanda did the practice, lifting her imaginary ax and bringing it down, I saw her anger and rage begin to boil. I encouraged her to keep going, and after about eight powerful chops, she stopped and looked at me. She had felt powerless and helpless for so long, and now she was vibrating with intensity.

"What are you chopping down, Wanda?"

"Shut up!" she barked back louder than I expected.

She kept going, moving through her rage and anger and whatever was in her imagination, breaking them up with her power, movement, and breath.

After a few minutes of chopping, she stopped; she was trembling. Her hands softened and dropped her imaginary ax. Wanda knelt down, unsure of what to do with the hurt and pain. I asked her to remove a large pillow from her couch and place it in front of her.

"Wanda, let's channel that anger and rage. I *invite* you to pound on the pillow."

She looked at me reluctantly, afraid she might look stupid.

I told her, "Let's take some time to release the anger. This is a place that doesn't need words. Just pound on the pillow. You choose the speed. It doesn't matter if it's fast or slow. The pillow can take it."

She pounded on the pillow slowly at first with her palms, then more powerfully with her fists (see Pounding Out, page 92).

"Give the pain a sound," I encouraged her. "Express it."

Wanda let out a deep painful cry. The cry of a daughter who missed her mom. The cry of years of repressed pain. An angry scream at God for the injustice. A cry of anger at the pandemic and for all those who failed to show up for her in her time of need.

At some point, she began to weep, and she collapsed in tears on the pillow. They were the tears of a daughter who couldn't get angry and who missed her mother.

What Wanda did isn't easy. Expressing who you are and how you feel takes deep courage. It feels like you are showing a wounded part of yourself. And yet when we acknowledge how we're wounded, it allows us to see how unique we are. This is what helps us to share what's important to us in life and in our heart.

Expressing who you are and how you feel takes deep courage.

LEARNING EXPRESSION

There are many ways we can feel stuck in expressing our emotions. One of the tools I incorporate in Grief Yoga is using sound, breath, and the vibration of the voice. Sometimes we may not always have the right words to express the reality of our struggle, but we need a way for it to be expressed so it can move through us. I often encourage my students to use their breath and voice to express and release the struggle.

When lions roar, they express not with words but with sound—and their message is heard. When cats meow, they communicate clearly whether they are hungry or want affection. When dogs bark, they communicate danger or warning. Animals can teach us to feel our feelings and express them, and then to let them go, shake them off, and move on. When my dog, Lucy, gets freaked out and scared, she feels it, expresses it, then moves forward to the next feeling.

What if people did that? Instead of suppressing our fears, what if we expressed them fully and then moved forward? Easier said than done, I know. We've been *taught* not to express certain feelings—and so we need to unlearn suppression and learn expression. Children also express their feelings freely, at least until they are taught not to. If children are sad, they cry. If they're angry, they throw a temper tantrum. Then they move forward. Of course, not every expression of emotion is appropriate. As adults, we know that kicking and screaming on the floor of the grocery store will not fix whatever has upset us. Adults don't do that— but they still might dump their unexpressed anger on the grocery store clerk for no reason. Sometimes, when we feel bad, we respond by making someone else feel bad, but this expression of suppressed emotions isn't any more appropriate than a tantrum.

Instead of suppressing our fears, what if we expressed them fully and then moved forward?

70

Thus, the challenge of adulthood is learning how to express challenging emotions in appropriate ways and at appropriate times, which is what Grief Yoga is all about.

When we express our challenging emotions about loss, we honor the loss that we've experienced. We own our feelings and express them in a way that is true. To discern if we are expressing emotions in appropriate or inappropriate ways, we can inquire within—are we being true to ourselves and in all areas of our lives? Are we expressing our anger and grief truthfully, or are we denying this important aspect of who we are? Expressing our truth about our grief and anger allows our pain to be witnessed. This is deeply important because our expression is a symbol of who we are. Grief matters because it is a symbol of love.

Often, it can be hard to know if we're being true to ourselves, as we can withhold our truths even from ourselves. Just remember that the body never lies. If you listen to your body, it will tell you what unresolved anger or sadness you may still be carrying, and the practice of Grief Yoga will help you release it, openly and honestly, so that you can move forward.

That's why I created this practice. So that we can dive deep into the shadow aspect of our sadness and anger, knowing that we will be okay. Through this work, we learn to love our shadow and allow ourselves the space to express our fears.

THE SPACE TO GRIEVE

My sister, Ella, died from cancer in 2017. Since her death, my mother has told me that she hasn't really expressed tears or sadness. When I was curious and asked her why, she said, "Well, I know she's in heaven. That is what we're told, and I believe it 100 percent. Why be sad?"

I believe Ella is in heaven, and she is no longer in pain. But there can still be sadness in that—the sadness of a mother grieving that she will never see her baby girl here on earth again. My mother, I believe, still feels that expressing sadness means that she is questioning her faith. I see the pain in her, but she won't speak of it. She needs to feel blessed and not have those negative feelings. But of course,

Jesus expressed his sadness. Jesus wept. Jesus showed and expressed his anger.

I told my mom about a dark night taking care of my sister in the hospital. Ella was deep in the throes of pain. Her stomach was bloated with waste and fluid due to a large cancerous tumor.

I wanted to do anything I could to help distract her from the pain. I placed my hands on her stomach and started gently rubbing. As she cried in pain, she kept saying, "It hurts. It hurts so much."

I tried anything I could to help her. I kept massaging her stomach in a clockwise motion. In Grief Yoga, I often have my students put their hands on their stomach and realize the power of their core. My sister couldn't do this for herself, but I could do it for her. Pain is a feeling that demands expression. By pushing as she requested, I was able to help her express that pain. She released it through sound, giving her pain a voice. I could help her to recognize her own strength. Every day of her illness, I observed her warrior-like power to look cancer in the face, though her body was so frail. I wanted her to see it, too.

"Where are you, Jesus?" Ella cried out. "Why aren't you here to help me? You said you were going to heal me!" Her tears shattered my heart.

"Let's be angry at God," I said to her. This took Ella aback. "God can take it," I insisted.

I let loose a primal roar and scream. Ella's eyes lit up. I did it again, a primal roar expressing my anger at life, suffering, and God. I wanted to make the voice of her pain louder, more powerful.

I looked at her and she let out a gut-wrenching scream and roar. It was her sound of fighting for her life as she pushed through this terrible pain.

We screamed these deep roars together.

Ella's frail body sat up. "I'm not the type of mother who will abandon her sons. That's not the mother I am."

Ella's three kids had spent most of their life knowing their mom as someone who was fighting cancer. She was fighting to stay alive for them.

I let out another primal roar like a lion, and she did the same. There was a moment of silence as we looked at one another, and then we laughed.

"Let's go for a walk," Ella said. I got her walker and placed it in front of her. I helped her fragile body get up as we slowly moved out of the room.

"You got this," she kept repeating to herself. "You got this." It sounded like she was forcing herself to believe it. I placed my hand on her bony back and took small steps with her.

"I got you, Ella. You're doing so good." As we walked under the bright lights of the hospital hallways, I kept thinking, *One small step at a time*. Walking with her made me think about how she knew she needed to move. Even in this weakness, she knew she couldn't just sit in her pain; she *had* to move forward even in these small steps. Movement is the core of Grief Yoga. All I could do for her, as I do for my students, was to help her move.

After about ten minutes, she whispered, "That's it. I gotta go back." We slowly headed back to her room. Ella asked me to play some music she had brought with her.

"Thank you, Jesus, for saving me," the woman sang. "Thank you, Jesus, for healing me." This filled my sister as she shifted back into her devotion. She had expressed her pain, and this spiritual song helped her connect to her healing.

EXPRESSION AS RELEASE

That experience with my sister taught me that anger can come and go, and sadness can come and go. When these feelings come, the only way to move through them is to express them, so you can truly feel them. You can do this in a variety of ways: through talking to a friend or counselor, journaling, writing letters that you don't intend to send, kickboxing, dancing, and of course yoga. When deciding what to do, or which specific Grief Yoga techniques to choose from, rely on your intuition, for that will guide you to *your* most authentic expression. This will be your most effective method for releasing your pain.

We all need to express our reality in our own way, and our bodies are the simplest tool. Our issues are in our tissues, and we need to let them out.

To process the pain of grief, you have to feel it. You can't heal what you don't feel. Feel *all* your feelings, the good and the bad. The exercises, techniques, and moving meditations provided in this chapter can help you access your emotions, but oftentimes feelings of grief come out of nowhere. When this happens, don't fight it. Let yourself just be with these emotions, letting them flow like ocean waves. Feel any disappointment, fear, or sadness. Connect to where you're feeling these emotions in your body. Allow yourself to react emotionally to your loss.

This is challenging, and it requires discipline—it's the act of igniting a fire within, so that we can reach our desired goal. We must force ourselves to go against the grain of learned habit. Sitting on your grief, keeping it hidden, can seem like the easier thing, but painful emotions will only keep you stuck. They require heat and light in order to be released. This is what the step of expression is for.

EXPRESSION TECHNIQUES AND EXERCISES

Wanda is an example of how to take challenging emotions like rage and suppressed pain and release them. Expressing emotions can feel embarrassing or pointless at first, but with practice it becomes incredibly liberating. You do not need to express your emotions to anyone other than yourself—all that is important is that these emotions are *felt*, as deeply as they are asking you to feel them.

The following exercises and practices guide your body through expressing your emotions, to release your struggle. Some of these will resonate while others may not. Explore and find what works for you.

Cannon Breath

This practice helps infuse your body with fresh oxygen, giving you energy, clearing out the stale air, and opening the throat to release your pain and express what you are experiencing. This practice externalizes your emotions, moving them out of you. You don't even have to clearly understand these emotions as they go—just move them along.

1. From a comfortable seated position, bring your fists to your belly and observe your natural breath.

2. Inhale three quick breaths through your nose and fill your diaphragm with air. As you breathe, you will literally feel the pressure build.

3. Next, in a powerful release, exhale strongly through your mouth, voicing a loud "HA!" Push your palms in toward your navel as you vocalize to clear out any stale oxygen as you open your throat.

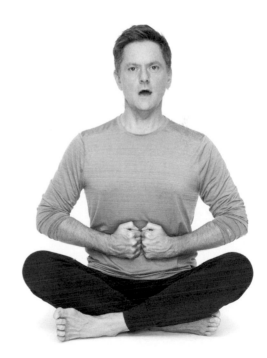

4. Continue for one minute, repeating this sequence at your own pace: Inhale three quick breaths through your nose, and exhale like a powerful cannonball breath through your mouth, voicing "HA!" The quick inhales force the spine to lengthen and straighten, while the powerful exhale creates a heavy sigh, releasing any stored emotions.

Breaking the Chains

When I teach this practice to bereavement groups or cancer-support centers, sometimes people say, "Since my loved one died, I haven't been able to laugh or cry for months. I feel confined, restrained." We *can* be free to laugh, to cry. We need not be constrained by grief, which is a free-flowing experience that should not be bound.

1. From a comfortable seated position, hold your arms in front of your chest, bent at the elbows, with one forearm on top of the other. Make tight fists with your hands, which sit at each elbow. Imagine and connect to where you're feeling stuck in your life and your struggle.

2. Inhale deeply, and as you exhale, push both elbows back with a powerful "HA!"

3. Continue for one to three minutes, repeating the sequence at your own pace. Connect to your roar as you exhale with a sharp "HA!" This releases where you feel stuck in your throat. As you push your elbows back, connect to your empowerment and open your heart.

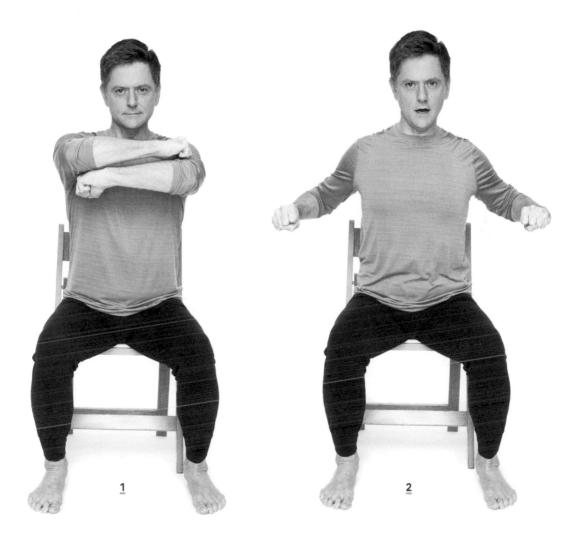

1   2

77

Punching Out

————

Grief is exhausting. We hold so much pain inside. This exercise encourages you to ignite and activate a spark within so you can channel and release anger and fear in empowering ways.

1. From a comfortable seated position, bring tight fists to your heart. Observe your breath and connect to any anger and frustration.

2. Begin to punch out in front of you, alternating fists. Choose your own speed and intensity, and maintain that momentum. As you punch, breathe either using quick inhalations and exhalations through your mouth or long deep breaths.

3. Continue for one to three minutes or for as long as you want. After you finish, come back to your natural breath.

HONOR YOUR ANGER

So much of grief is clouded by anger. This is natural—and it is natural not to want to let go of that anger, since it can feel like a form of protection from sadness. Anger is often sadness's bodyguard, but we can fear unleashing anger, since it might be too much. What if we hurt someone? If we keep it in, it might. Misplaced anger is hard for loved ones to take. But when we honor the anger and let it move through, it has the space to run its course and is less likely to get released on the wrong people.

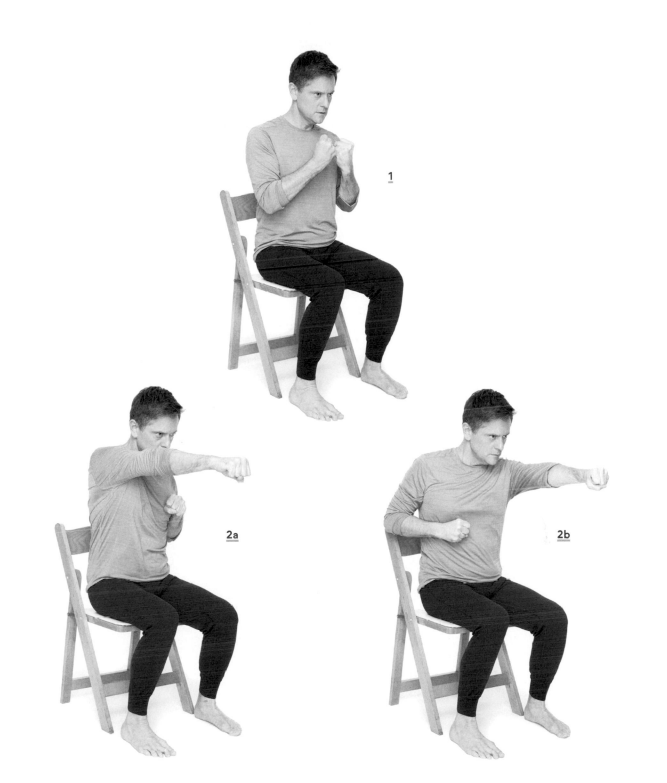

Woodchopper

The Woodchopper creates the space to release anger and rage. As you embrace any feelings of being betrayed, insulted, or abandoned, you can feel your pent-up rage gathering force. Unleash it so it doesn't burn you up inside. Be big with this gesture. Embody your defiance.

1. Stand with your feet hip-width apart and your knees slightly bent.

2. Bring your hands together, interlace your fingers, and raise your arms up over your head.

3. With elbows straight, bend forward and bring your arms down hard while yelling "HA!" as loudly as you can. This activates your energy center while you release tension and anger with your breath and the vibration of your voice.

4. Continue for as long as you wish, repeating the sequence at your own pace. Vocalize as loudly as you can. Move through whatever is weighing you down. When you feel that the anger or rage has left your body, stand softly, close your eyes, breathe, and feel.

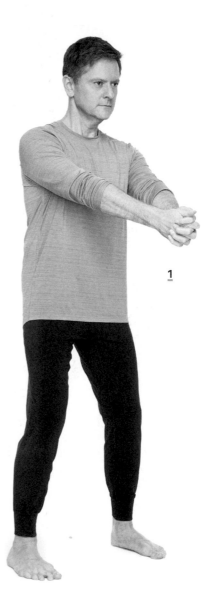

1

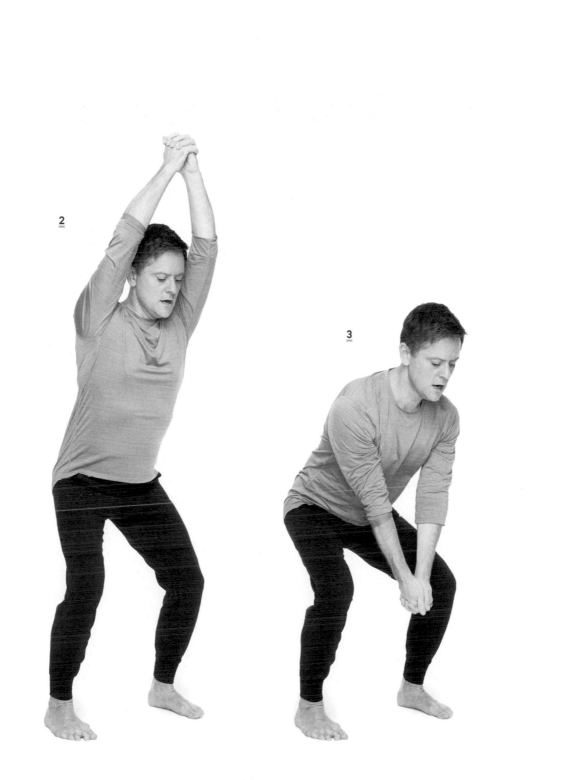

Releasing the Why

When we are faced with the biggest, most confusing, and horrific events that could ever happen, we often ask why. While we have a right to ask that question, we may not get a full answer, or any answer at all, and part of our task is to learn to live with what can't be known. This technique will help you move through that process.

1. From a standing position, take a step forward with one leg, lift your arms up, palms facing toward you, and say loudly, "Why?"

2. Come back to a neutral standing position and repeat, using the other leg: Step, reach upward, and exclaim, "Why?"

3. Continue at your own pace for one to three minutes, or for as long as you want. Keep alternating legs, and vary your vocalizations; whisper or scream. If you want, gaze up as you ask, "Why?"

EXPRESSING "WHY?"

Why did they die? Why now? Why them? Why me?

In grief, we have a primal need to ask why. We may direct this question at God, at the person who has died, or at ourselves—or all of the above.

Sometimes it is impossible to know why something happened, and friends and relatives may tell us to stop asking, but that doesn't make the need to know go away. Although we may never discover the reason for loss and pain, expressing "Why?" can help us to move through the struggle.

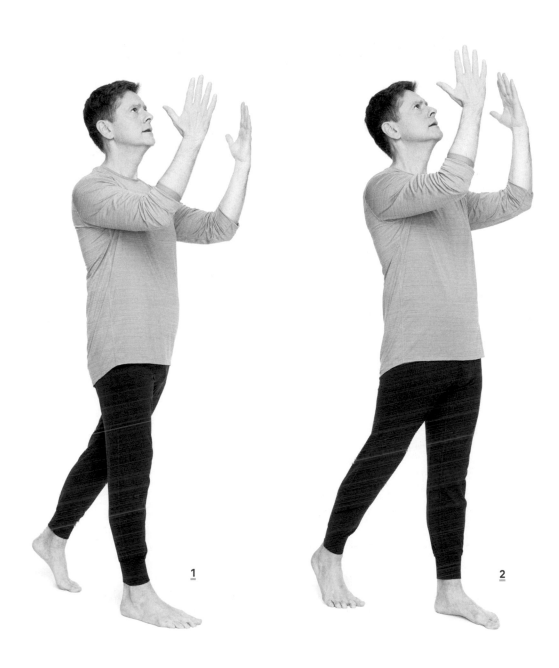

Windmill

Sometimes our feelings can be so overwhelming it's hard to breathe. We may not have the words to articulate these feelings, but you can release them with movement, breath, and sound. This cleansing exercise allows you to discharge those unnamed feelings, to express and release them using your breath, body, and the vibration of your voice, without requiring words you may not be able to find.

1. From a neutral standing position, feet hip-width apart, knees slightly bent, inhale as you lift your hands up over your head. As you do, breathe in any tension, anxiety, or feelings of being overwhelmed as you open the front line of your body.

2. As you exhale, bend your upper body forward, hinging from your hips, and letting your arms release to swing forward, down, and behind you. As your arms swing, use your breath and the vibration of your voice to discharge and release your emotions, flinging them away.

3. As you inhale, bring your arms back up and return to a standing position, with your arms over your head. Again, breathe in any tension or anxiety.

4. Again, as you exhale, hinge forward, knees bent, letting your arms swing and fall, and vocalize as you release behind you any struggle.

5. Continue at your own pace for two minutes.

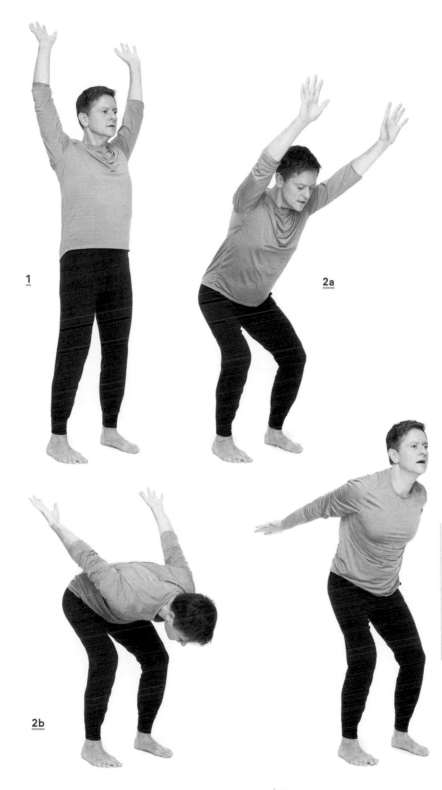

1

2a

2b

VARIATION

If bending forward at the waist is uncomfortable, remain standing, and as you exhale, let your arms swing forward, down, and behind you.

Clearing the Path

In our life path, we encounter many stumbling blocks along the way. Obstacles like doubt, shame, unhealthy habits, limiting beliefs, and negative situations or circumstances can get in our way and keep us from moving forward. Perhaps we believe that we failed or did something wrong. It can be liberating to remove judgments that drain our energy. This empowering technique suggests holding imaginary divine swords that aren't meant to hurt or harm; they help chop and clear away obstacles, like machetes, so you can move forward.

1. From a seated or standing position, with your feet hip-width apart, raise both hands out to your sides and make fists, as if you were holding imaginary divine swords.

2. Inhale and reach one arm up toward your opposite shoulder. Exhale and move your arm in a chopping motion diagonally in front of you. Inhale and move your other hand to your opposite shoulder; on the exhale chop your arm swiftly and powerfully across your body.

3. Keep alternating arms and using imaginary swords to cut away any struggle or obstacle holding you back. As you do, voice a powerful "HA!" to empower you.

4. Continue at your own pace for one to three minutes, then release your imaginary swords and come back to your natural breath.

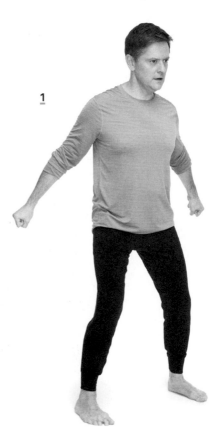

1

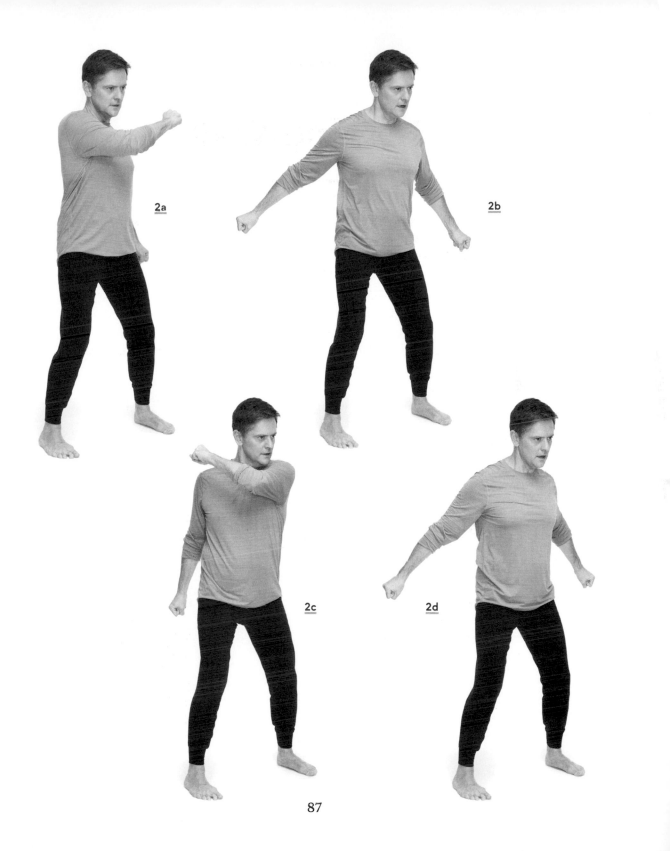

2a

2b

2c

2d

87

Kicking Out

In grief, we can feel like we're trapped in a box. Our grief envelops us, and we wonder if we'll ever get out. Kicking out at that pain helps us to get our space back. We need to tap into whatever power we can, and our legs have power. Embracing the power in your legs helps you to unleash yourself. Your anger helps you break out of the confined box of pain.

1. Assume a tabletop position on your hands and knees, with your shoulders over your hands and your hips over your knees. Do a light shakeout, releasing any tension.

2. As you inhale, bring one knee in toward your nose as you round your back.

    VARIATION

    For better support, feel free to place a pillow under your knees and place your forearms on the ground.

3. As you exhale, kick the leg back with a powerful "HA!" Release any pain, hurt, or struggle. You can choose how quickly or slowly to kick. Repeat this sequence with the same leg for one minute.

4. Switch to the other leg. Inhale and bring the other knee in toward your nose, and as you exhale, kick back with a powerful "HA!" Repeat with the same leg for a minute, releasing and moving through any frustration and pain.

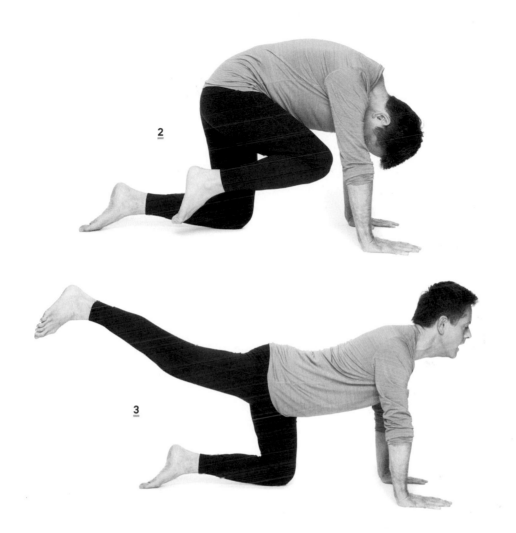

RELEASE DISAPPOINTMENT

This practice may start with expressing anger, but be aware that it may end in tears. It might turn into rage that needs to be released. You may find that as you dive deeper into your anger, you move beyond it into sadness and disappointment—sadness for your loved one who has died, and disappointment in any friends or family who may not have been there for you as you might have wished. Know that this is normal, and this is a safe way to feel and express that disappointment.

Defying Loss

———

This practice gives you permission to lie on the floor like an enraged toddler and throw a tantrum. Yes, you get to do that! You have *reasons* to be this angry. Your anger isn't wrong or unjust. You get to have your anger. Embrace it and feel it fully.

1. Lie on your back on the mat and lift your legs toward the sky. Or if you prefer, bend your knees and leave your feet on the ground.

2. With your hands at your sides, palms facing down, pound on the mat with your palms, releasing all your frustration and anger as you do.

3. Add your voice—scream out your frustrations as your anger releases.

4. Continue for as long as you wish. When you're ready, rest on your back. Bring one hand to your belly and the other to your heart. Surrender to stillness as you observe your breath.

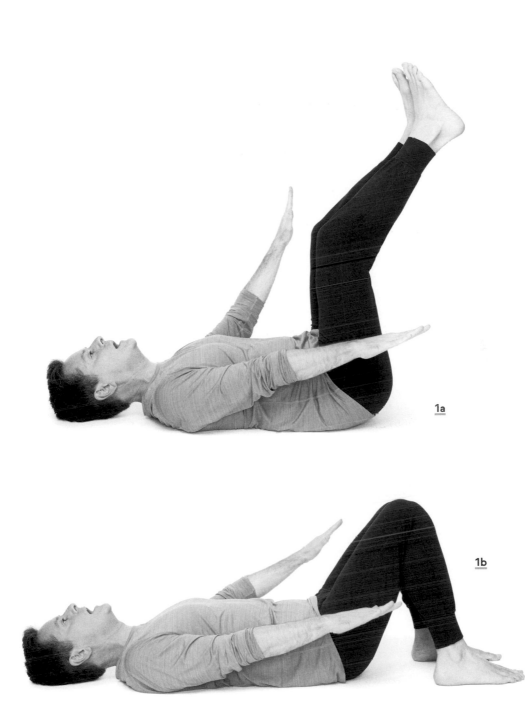

1a

1b

Pounding Out

———

We all have anger that we don't want to talk about. This exercise provides a space for what is unspoken.

1. From a comfortable kneeling position, place a pillow in front of you.

2. In whatever manner you wish, hit or pound the pillow continuously, using your fists to express and release any anger or resentment. You may initially feel reluctance, but keep going, choosing the speed that's right for you, whether fast or slow.

3. As you do this, use your voice, breath, and sound to release and discharge any jealousy or rage. Use words or simply scream a powerful or prolonged "HA!"

4. Continue pounding for as long as you want. The pillow can take it. When you feel finished, collapse onto your pillow. As you lie on the floor, feel whatever you're feeling and breathe deeply.

RELEASE RESENTMENTS

Sometimes our anger can feel wrong, even to us—we recognize that it can be socially unacceptable. For instance, it's not unusual for a widow or widower to be jealous of happily married couples. It's not unusual for bereaved parents to be resentful of those who have healthy, living children. When parents die young, surviving children can resent those who still have their parents. These jealous rages are often unspoken, but that doesn't mean they don't exist. They are perfectly understandable reactions to grief, and behind closed doors, I hear people express these "unacceptable" feelings all the time. Pounding Out is designed to let you give voice to that jealous rage.

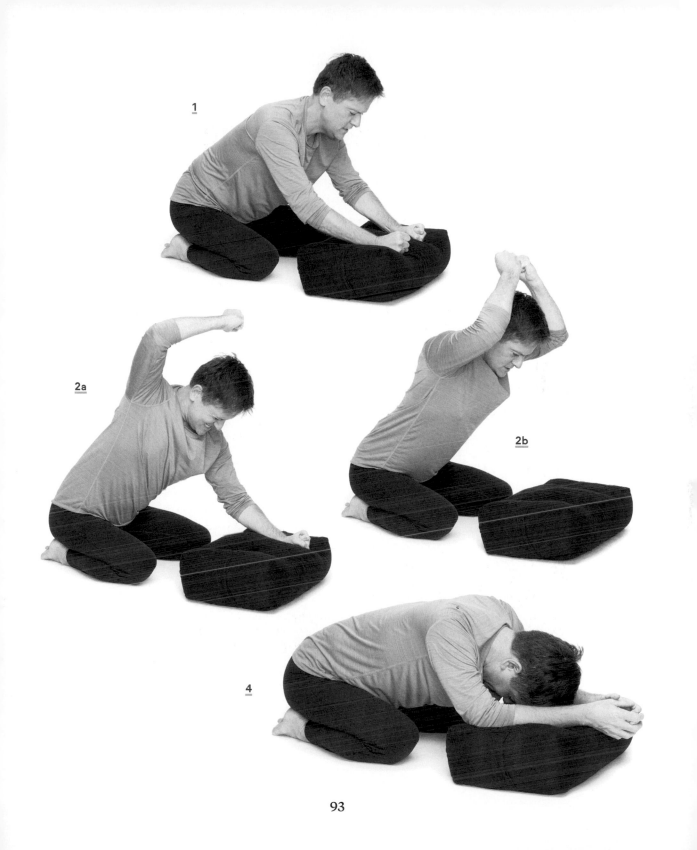

1

2a

2b

4

93

Releasing Pain

——

This practice is about letting go. It's about releasing the situation, releasing the hurt, releasing what was and no longer is. Release the pain of separation, the pain of watching a loved one become sick and die. We have to move that pain out of us. We must say goodbye to the life we planned with them. This practice helps to express and release that pain and hurt.

1. From a comfortable seated position, bring both hands in tight fists to your heart, elbows by your sides, and breathe deeply. Connect to where you hold any struggle in your life, mind, or body. Connect to your grief, your pain, your anger, your frustration—everything that you have been feeling.

2. Inhale deeply, and as you exhale, push one hand forward, open your fingers, and use your breath and a loud vocalization to discharge the pain and let it move through you. Use a powerful sound or word, such as "No," "Out," or "HA!" Let this feel primal, representing pain beyond words, and visualize the pain moving from your heart and out through your fingertips.

3. Inhale and bring your arm back, clenching two tight fists to your heart. As you exhale, extend the other hand in the same manner, vocalizing and releasing pain through your hand and breath.

4. Continue this sequence at your own pace for one to three minutes, or for as long as you wish. Alternate arms and build momentum. Welcome the new energy this creates and allow it to move through you. Release and let it go.

5. When you feel finished, or when you've channeled your pain through, sit quietly and breathe deeply until you feel grounded. You may feel energized by this momentum or you may feel drained from the release.

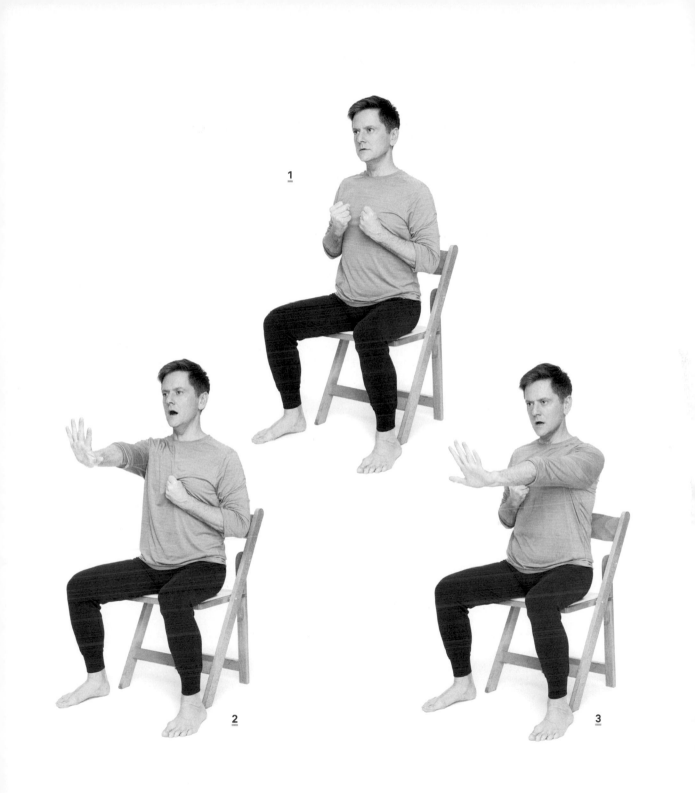

Pulling Up the Weeds

———

The purpose of this exercise is to bring to awareness any subconscious or repressed thoughts and unresolved feelings related to grief. As these come up, simply be aware and open to whatever arises, and acknowledge any regrets, guilt, blame, and doubts. Releasing unresolved emotions related to the past allows us to find more peace in the present and to learn to trust the process of life again after loss.

1. From a comfortable seated position, breathe. As you do, consider your loss and any unresolved feelings or regrets you may have. Ask yourself, *What if . . . ?* What comes to mind, or how would you complete that sentence?

2. When you identify a specific thought, inhale, and imagine that thought as a weed that you hold in one of your hands in front of you.

3. As you exhale, throw the weed over your head behind you, releasing the thought and letting it go, and bring your hand down to your side.

4. Then ask yourself again, *What if . . . ?* Or complete sentences that begin with "I should have" or "If only I had." When you identify another thought, imagine it as a weed you hold in front of you in the other hand. Inhale, and as you exhale, throw the weed over your head, release the thought, let it go, and bring your hand down by your side.

5. Continue this sequence, alternating hands, for three to five minutes, or for as long as you wish. Keep identifying specific regrets and unresolved feelings related to the loss and those involved; acknowledge each thought, throw it away, and let it go. When you're finished, sit quietly and come back to your breath.

VARIATION

You can also focus this practice on regrets related to other people. Finish the sentences "You should have," "If only you had," and "What if you did."

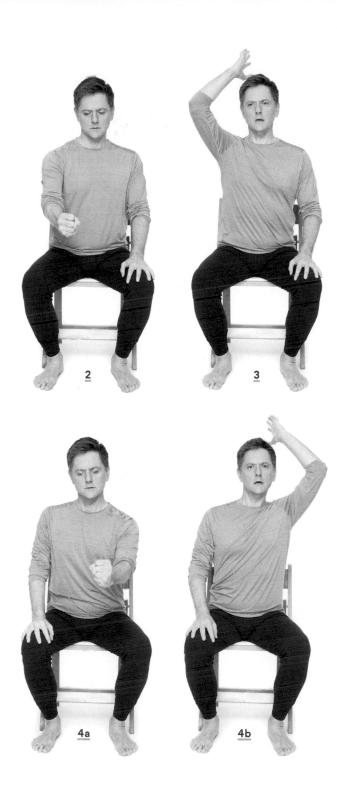

2

3

4a

4b

UPROOT REGRETS

"What ifs," "should haves," and "if onlys" are weeds of regret that foster doubt and stand in the way of fully embodying our grief. They are often ways we assign blame: "If only we had gone to another hospital," "What if they had tried another round of chemo," "I should have picked up the phone." The sad yet peaceful reality is that, despite what we or others might have done differently, our loved one would likely have died anyway. By pulling up these weeds after a loss, we release ourselves from feeling stuck in regret, doubt, guilt, and sadness so we can move through our grief.

Throwing Out the Struggle

———

This exercise is similar to Releasing Pain, but it focuses on our struggles when experiencing grief. For instance, other people can sometimes say stupid, thoughtless things, like, "Move on," "You can get another husband," "God never gives us more than we can handle." Also, we might struggle with normal life, which isn't normal anymore, such as a widow eating dinner alone. Acknowledge whatever your struggle is, and for now—just throw it out.

1. Stand with your feet parallel and hip-width apart, with knees slightly bent and your hips low.

2. Bring your hands to your heart and make tight fists. Observe your breath, and connect to any pain and struggle you feel.

3. Inhale deeply, and on the exhale, throw both hands out, to your side and behind you, spread your fingers, and exclaim, "Out," "Enough," or simply, "HA!" With this gesture, release the struggle and throw it away.

4. As you inhale, bring your fists back to your chest, and on the exhale, repeat the gesture, throwing your hands out behind you, releasing the emotions with your breath, and vocalizing powerfully.

5. Continue this sequence at your own pace for one to two minutes, or until you feel that you have thrown away everything that's keeping you in a place of struggle and suffering.

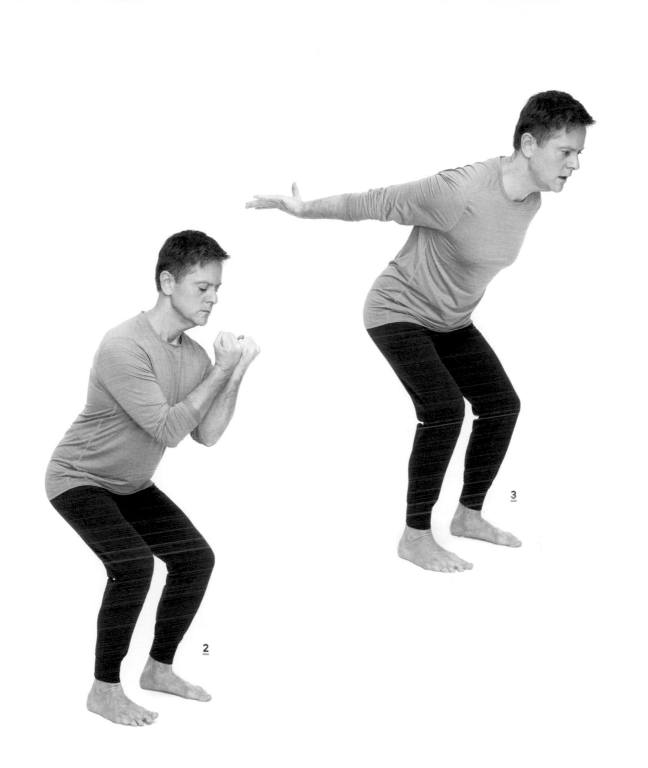

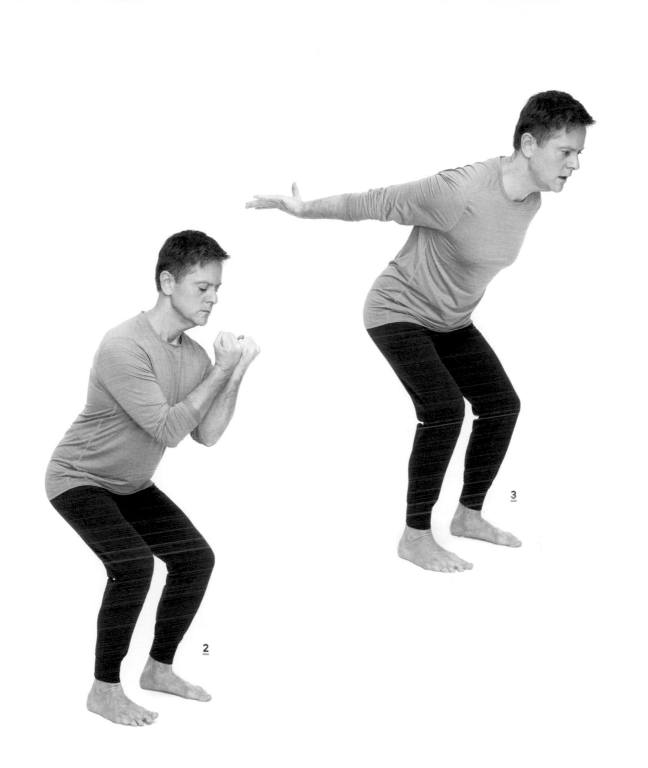 2

3

99

Shake It

―――

No one can sit in pain all the time—at a certain point, we have to release it, just for a moment, knowing and trusting that it won't go away. Remember, shaking off your pain does not mean shaking off the memory of your loved one. You are shaking off all the other stuff that covers and clouds the love you have for that person.

1. From a comfortable seated or standing position, simply shake out your hands and release whatever you're carrying or feeling, whatever is keeping you in a place of struggle. Just shake it off.

2. Continue shaking your hands for as long as you want, or as long as feels necessary. If you wish, also shake your arms, shoulders, head, and entire body.

3. Another variation is to play an energetic song that gets your whole body moving. Don't even think about it. Just move organically to the music and rhythm and have some fun with it. Keep moving until everything feels shaken off.

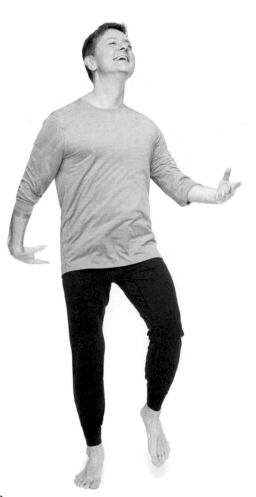

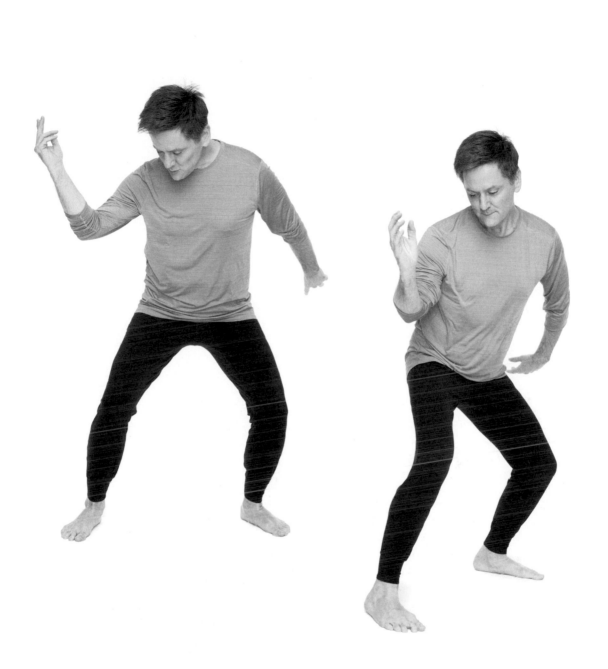

Continues

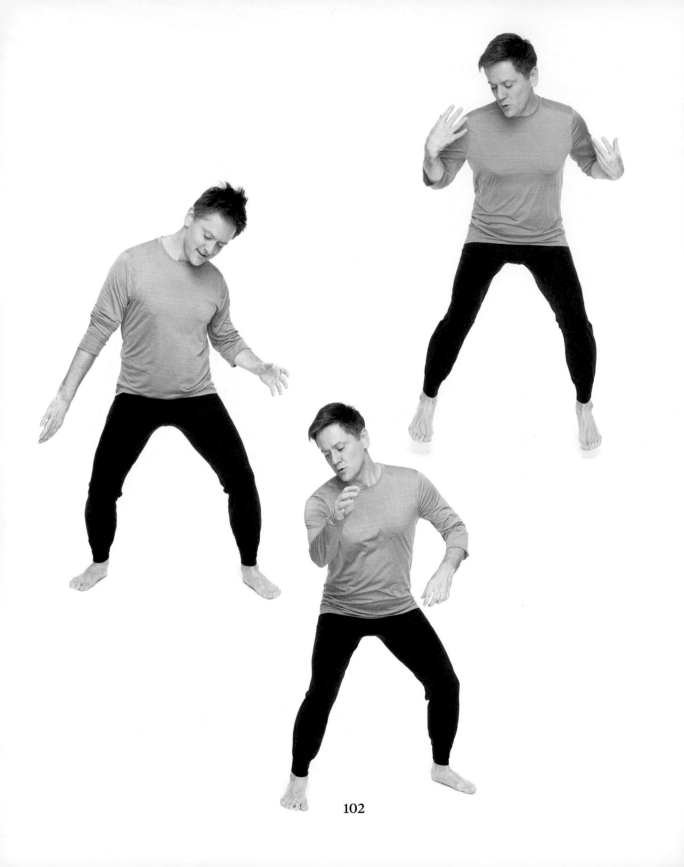

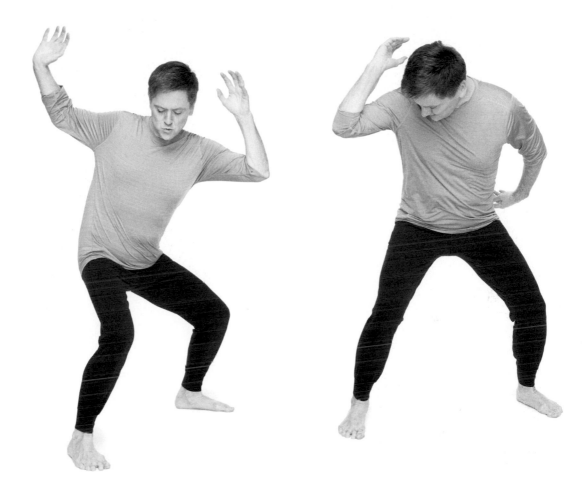

Moving into Connection

Expression can be draining. At the end of these exercises, you may feel tired, even exhausted. That's not only normal, it's a good thing. When you've emptied yourself of pain and struggle, you've made space for a new way of being with your grief. Connection guides you into that space, as you rediscover self-love, compassion, and kindness.

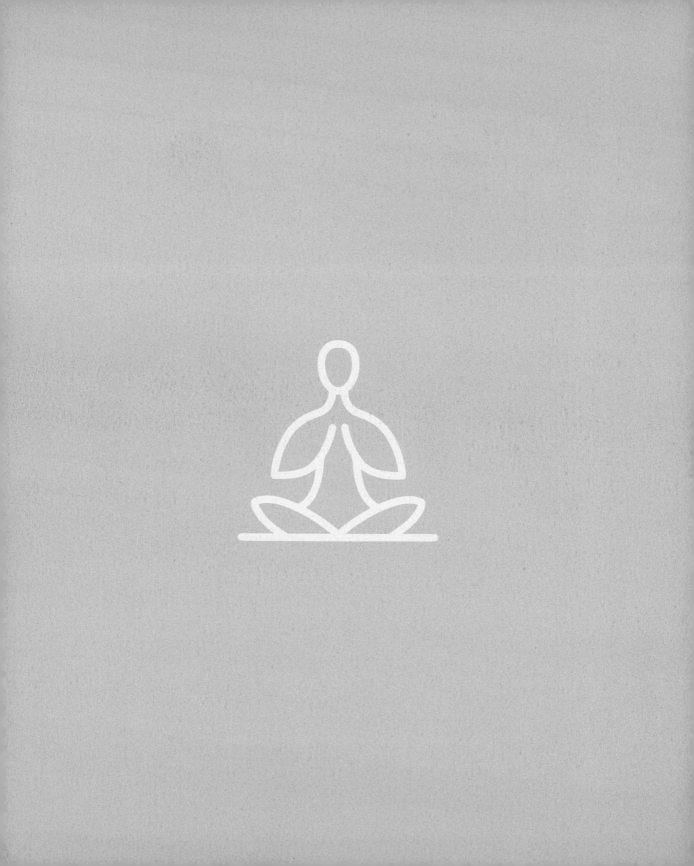

3

Connection

There are no goodbyes for us. Wherever you are,
you will always be in my heart.

—MAHATMA GANDHI

Connection helps to ease the suffering of feeling separated. Whether that connection happens within yourself, with another, or through spirit, it's a path toward more love, grace, and gratitude.

Once you've expressed your struggle, you can begin to shift your pattern and allow a different flow, one that moves toward connection. The root of suffering is disconnection. We feel grief because we are literally disconnected from someone or something that we love. This disconnection is inevitable—one day, we will lose the people we love, one way or another. Grief is a part of this life experience.

When our physical connection is gone, we don't know what to do with the energy that remains. Our grief is love that doesn't know where to go. But we can still send our love to the person who has died. We knew how to love them when they were present; now we must love them in their absence.

You can find connection again within yourself, with another person who is still living, or through a deeper spiritual connection with your loved one who has died. That can look different for everyone, but finding connection again will guide you to a deeper place of gratitude and appreciation of your life.

For me, I deeply miss my sister, Ella. I deeply miss beloved friends. I deeply miss my buddy and doggy companion, Angel.

In those moments of disconnection, I close my eyes. I see them in my mind's eye, and I connect to the love I feel for them still. As tears begin to flow, I whisper to them, "I'm sending you love. I'm thinking of you and sending you love." I have no idea if they know or are receiving my love, but I believe they are. It eases my heart and mind. I can still love them, and sending them love allows the love a place to go: "Thank you for the love you gave me. Thank you for making my life more meaningful. Thank you for breaking my heart with your absence because I see and feel what's important in life."

This is connection, which is what Grief Yoga guides us toward.

FINDING CONNECTION

Sometimes, you need to plug into something greater than yourself to connect with the energy and gift of life.

I remember the first time my student Jaquelin attended one of my yoga classes. Some people just catch your attention. Jaquelin was in her late thirties, a tall, powerful woman with a sparkle in her eyes. She beamed kindness, and her smile was playful and mischievous. She blended strength and softness. Jaquelin taught me about connecting to spirit through movement. She was a movement and dance teacher, and when she danced, she flowed like the wind, embodying the movement of a powerful goddess. Or she moved with the rhythmic intensity of a fiery tornado or the gentle sway of a protective, caring mother. She taught me about the pleasures and joy that can be found in dance, and how it can be a tool for healing.

One day Jaquelin was sick and had to cancel her dance class. There was a flu going around. No big deal, right? It happens all the time. A week later, the next thing I heard, she was in the ER. I thought it must be a bad flu, and I was surprised, considering how healthy she was.

Three days later, I got the call that Jaquelin had died. It seemed impossible. Not her, not someone so vital, so young. We all know that people die from the normal, everyday flu, which goes around every year, but how could Jaquelin be one of them? At forty-three, she was gone, and the community she created didn't know what to do.

When she died, shock waves rippled through me and our community. How could someone so healthy and strong die suddenly? We lost our connection to so much joy, so much pleasure, and so much loving support. However, it's possible to restore and re-create that connection, at least within ourselves. Today, when I want to remember

Sometimes, you need to plug into something greater than yourself to connect with the energy and gift of life.

Jaquelin and reflect on the gifts she gave me, I play a song that she often danced to, Nat King Cole's "Unforgettable." Then, with my eyes closed, I remember how she danced and I move that way myself. I feel like she has joined me and her spirit is dancing with me (see Dance Prayer, page 144).

Life is filled with so much struggle. And as much as, through Grief Yoga, I want to honor grief, anger, and struggle, Jaquelin taught me to honor love, laughter, and pleasure. We shouldn't forget these colors of life. To keep Jaquelin's memory alive, I remind myself that it's important to take time to embrace pleasure, whether that's through movement, eating a delicious piece of cake, watching the sunset, or listening to the birds sing just because they're alive. When I find a moment that brings me pleasure, I know she would approve.

"Connect to this gift of life, Paul," I remember her saying. "Enjoy the simple pleasures in life. And flow in your own unique way. You come from a long line of ancestors and those who came before you. Perhaps they're supporting you here now."

I feel Jaquelin's spiritual presence with me now, connecting with me in this moment. Even though I want to have her here physically, to hug her and see her nurturing smile, I connect to her spirit and the memories we shared together.

PATHS TOWARD CONNECTION

There are three paths in Grief Yoga that embrace connection: love, gratitude, and grace.

Connecting with Love

If I am fully aware and can express myself, I can connect with all the sides of myself—and I can choose to love them. I can choose to love my sadness, my lack of trust, my pain, my hurt, my anger and disdain, my guilt, my shame. In this moment, I breathe. I place my hand on my heart. And I choose to love. I soften my mind and heart to love.

What if you loved all parts of yourself? Your shame, your stinginess, your anger? What if you loved even these aspects, as though they were an innocent, crying child you hold in your arms? Can you offer the love of kindness and compassion? Can you offer a caring blessing to the pain?

When I honor Jaquelin through a flowing meditation, I am moving out of love for her. This is my way of connecting with her, even though she is no longer moving. As I move in the ways she did, that movement is a devotion of love. It's a body prayer, saying, "Thank you for touching my heart." A whisper to her saying, "I love you. Thank you for loving me."

> Love is eternal. It was here before you arrived, and it will be here when you are gone.

Love is eternal. It was here before you arrived, and it will be here when you are gone. Can you be present to it while you're alive? Can you be present to it even after someone you loved is gone? They no longer exist but love always exists. Love never dies. Love is constantly surrounding you. In life, and in death. When people die, David Kessler says, "we don't stop loving them. And even in their death, they don't stop loving us."

That love continues. It can feel like our loved ones died and our connection with them is over, but this is not true. That relationship continues because the love never disappears.

Connecting with Gratitude

What if you were grateful for everything—not just the good or great things, but *everything,* even the pain? This isn't easy to do, but what if you could thank the struggle and pain? They can help you witness the fragility of life. Thank others for their gift of love and for breaking your heart. Both help us to feel and love deeply. In the midst of these feelings, we recognize we're alive. The buffet of life includes many emotions, and I'm grateful to feel all of them—the sadness, the grief, the joy, the love.

A woman named Carol once reached out to me to schedule an in-person session. As I walked up to her front door, I couldn't help but notice a beautiful willow tree that hung over her house as if it were protecting her from the light and from storms. As Carol answered the door, she smiled in greeting, but her smile didn't reach her eyes.

When someone we love dies, we are all left with bad memories.

"Thank you for visiting," she said. "My son died a few years ago, and I feel like I've done a lot of work around his death, but I'm curious about your practice." Carol described how she had witnessed her fourteen-year-old son, Jeremy, battling cancer for the last few years of his life through multiple hospitalizations. "I should have been able to save him," she said. "I have so many bad memories of those struggles."

I shared with her David Kessler's grief work and talked about his book *Finding Meaning*. When David became a bereaved father, he also felt, like nearly every parent he counsels, that he had failed in some way by not being able to save his son. David believes there is an unconscious belief parents have that success means keeping your child alive, and Carol perked up as she realized she was not alone in her pain.

She said, "The bad memories can be like an ongoing nightmare."

When someone we love dies, we are all left with bad memories. Once, when David and I were teaching at a weekend retreat, someone asked him if he had found gratitude. He said that it took time, but eventually he thought there was a tragedy worse than his son dying, which would be never having met his son in this lifetime.

Carol and I started our Grief Yoga class. I had her warm up with some awareness techniques to deepen her breath and move her body, and then we did some powerful expression techniques to move through any regrets she was holding.

I asked Carol, "Would you like to try a technique that might help you take in more of the good memories?" She nodded. I asked her to do the Appreciation Meditation (page 124). With her eyes closed and her empty hands in front of her—which reflected how she was feeling, empty and unsure of how to move forward—I asked her to visualize an experience she had shared with her son that she appreciated, that she was grateful for. Once she saw it, I asked her to say yes to it and bring her hands to her heart, holding that moment close for as long as she wanted while simply breathing and listening to her heartbeat. When she was ready, she brought her hands back out, ready to receive another memory.

Carol told me that until we worked together that day, she had no idea how much pain and regret she was still holding on to. She had been carrying the weight of believing that maybe if she had done something more, Jeremy would still be with her. But now she understood that, although her mind told her this, her heart didn't believe it was true. The doctors and nurses had called her Tiger Mama, and she knew she had done everything she could to help save her baby boy.

Focusing on gratitude helps us shift so that we remember our love. Our loved ones have a deep impact on our lives. They touch us in ways that will live in our hearts forever, creating a connection that cannot be lost.

It takes time to find gratitude in grief. You don't feel it for a long time, but it's there waiting for you. Gratitude isn't so much a feeling we experience—it's a decision we make. It's a way of looking at the world. The decision to be grateful is a path that can lift your mind and heart. It allows you to connect with your own life, with the life you share with others, and with the larger experience of the unknown that allows you to remain in relationship with those who have passed. We can be grateful for the time we've had with our loved ones.

Make a decision to appreciate life—including the boredom, the grief, the pain, the hurt. Appreciation is a continuous practice that reminds me I am a life force that feels deeply, and I'm thankful for that. I'm breathing. I'm still alive.

Allow yourself to choose gratitude. Take time to stop and observe. Look around and see everything in your life—the positive and the negative—and express

Allow yourself to choose gratitude. Take time to stop and observe.

thanks for it. Thank you for this home. Thank you for this dog. Thank you for these friends. Thank you for the sunshine and the rain. Thank you for my partner. Thank you for my job and work. Thank you for this body, with all its injuries. Decide to be grateful, even for that which is most challenging, and give thanks.

Connecting with Grace

Grace can grow in the midst of devastation. It's a companion within you, and it allows you to feel *all* of life's experiences, the joy with your grief, and everything else that comes. It helps you connect to the pain, the love, the laughter, the struggle.

For me, grace feels like a presence, like the presence of a parent behind their child who is learning to ride a bicycle. They hold and support the child as they move forward, until they let go. And yet they're still there.

Grace can be like a mother nurturing a child. When we're in the depths of despair, grace is the blanket that keeps us warm. Grace is a divine motherly presence that loves us unconditionally. She tells us, *You matter. Your love matters. Your grief matters.* And in the space when we feel like all is lost, that eternal mother of grace reminds us that this pain too shall pass.

Grace is something we receive, and it is something we give—and in the giving, we are also the recipients of grace. Forgiveness is an important aspect of grace, a medicine for the soul that heals both the forgiven and the one who forgives. If I am forgiven, then I am receiving grace, and if I forgive, I am giving *and* receiving grace because forgiveness is a kindness to ourselves.

This is a lifelong process. Forgiving others for their wrongs. Forgiving ourselves for all the mistakes we've made.

This is a lifelong process. Forgiving others for their wrongs. Forgiving ourselves for all the mistakes we've made. Forgiving what we didn't do and what we did do. Forgiving others and ourselves for our imperfections.

Forgiveness is possible in any moment. If you're having trouble reaching forgiveness with someone, try this: Picture the person as a baby, born innocent. This is how we all begin, and a baby can be forgiven anything—they know not what they do. Then watch them grow. Imagine their family dynamics and see how this baby must have been changed for them to become the person who could harm you in this way. Know that they were wounded, and that wounded people wound people. There is a grace in acknowledging someone's hurts as well as your own.

All forgiveness requires is willingness. It's a decision that we make to heal the hurt. It's not an easy decision to make, and sometimes, depending on the circumstances, it may feel impossible for us personally. We might not ever find the willingness to forgive someone. Yet it's still important to reach peace, to reach grace.

When we cannot forgive someone ourselves, we can reach grace by turning forgiveness over to God. We can allow ourselves to say, it is not our place to forgive this person—that is for God to do. We can decide to find peace by turning forgiveness over to God, and allowing the forgiveness of God is an act of grace.

CONNECTION TECHNIQUES AND EXERCISES

When dealing with loss, it's normal to feel disconnected and yearn for the love that is gone. Separation and disconnection can weigh heavy on us. In these moments of sadness and vulnerability, it's important to take care of yourself. The following techniques are ways to find connection through love, gratitude, and grace. Explore and find the ones that work for you.

Love for Ourselves

———

Grief lives in our body. Our body remembers the pain. This practice of self-embrace connects you to the love within and helps you embrace where you're wounded. The feeling of self-touch can be nourishing as you soothe tension with a shoulder massage and embrace. This is how we cultivate compassion and kindness for ourselves.

1. From a comfortable seated position, observe your natural breath. Place your hands on your body where you hold pain—your heart, hips, head, shoulders, and so on. Investigate and place your hands where pain lives in your body.

2. As you place your hands, compassionately connect to that part of your body and whisper, "I love you." If your hand is on your heart, send love to the sadness in your heart. Whisper, "My heart, I love you." Love your grief. Love the physical manifestation of it in your body. If your hand is on your head, whisper, "My head, I love you." Love the wound that is inside of you.

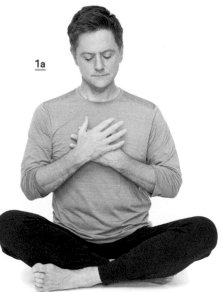

1a

3. You can also offer yourself a caring massage to soothe any tension. Or wrap your arms around your chest in an embrace, as if giving yourself a hug. Or bring one hand to the opposite shoulder, and the other hand to the other shoulder. Offer yourself love.

4. Continue for two to five minutes, breathing deeply and embracing yourself in this gentle meditation.

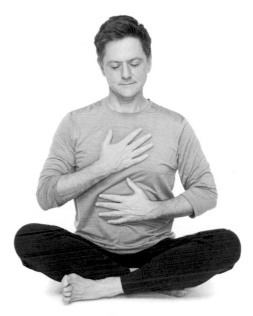

1b

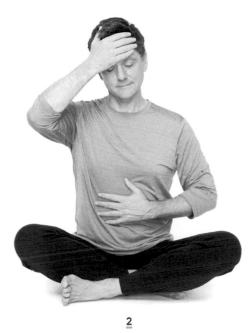

2

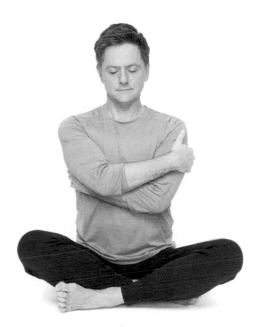

3a

3b

115

Cradling the Child

This is an invitation to be present and caring to the innocence within. By gently rocking, we connect to a gentle loving part of ourselves that can nurture and cradle us in times of sadness. Embrace this comforting motion and send love to the child within, who may be feeling lost, alone, afraid, or sad.

1. From a comfortable seated position, cradle your arms in front of your chest, palms facing up, as if you were holding an infant child in front of your heart.

2. Gently rock from side to side and breathe. Quietly send love to your child within, the innocent child you remember from long ago. Imagine nurturing this vulnerable child, and think or gently whisper, "I love you."

3. Continue this comforting cradle from side to side for one to four minutes.

WITNESS SADNESS

There are times when I don't know how to be with my sadness. It's too much, too overwhelming. And in those moments, I close my eyes and place my hand on my heart. I imagine myself as a little boy, lost, alone, and too afraid to show how sad he's feeling. In that sadness, as I witness that sad little boy, I say to him, "I'm with you now. I love you just as you are." That's connection within.

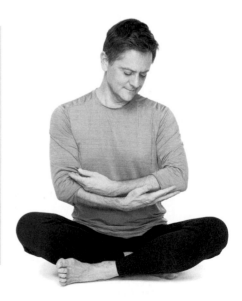

Love Taps

———

Unwitnessed grief can weigh heavy on our heart. It's normal to want to hide away and not let anyone see our pain. But once we acknowledge it and feel connected to ourself, we can find healing.

Witnessing your grief isn't about trying to find a solution. It's a technique to breathe, feel, express, and support yourself, a compassionate space to connect to your vulnerability, where your true strength lives.

1. From a comfortable seated position, lightly tap the tops of your fingertips on your chest and heart.

2. As you lightly tap your chest, connect to how your heart is feeling. As you tap, say, "I am . . . ," and complete the sentence with whatever your heart needs to share. It could be, "I am sad," "I am overwhelmed," or "I am scared." Whatever you're feeling, tap to connect to it and witness it. The only way out of the pain is to acknowledge it and move through it. Do this for one to three minutes.

3. When this feels complete, place your hands on your chest and heart and breathe. Hold the space where grief lives within you with loving tenderness. Connect to the resilient wiser part of you that guides you and imagine it speaking these words: *Let me take care of you. Let me sit with you in your sadness. Let me mend your heart because your beloved has died. When your heart is aching for what you've lost, I will help you move through the storm. When you are lonely and sad and longing for the past, I will open your heart and help you connect to that beautiful vulnerability within. Let me express that longing for your love.*

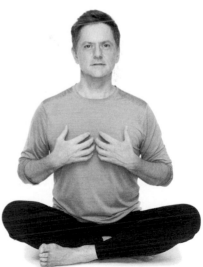

4. Hold your hands to your heart for one to three minutes. Then bring your hands to your sides and breathe deeply.

Holding Love

We never stop giving or receiving love, but we don't always realize it. There are many obstacles that can keep us disconnected from feeling this love that surrounds us: fear, shame, guilt, resentments, and so on. This moving meditation allows you to release these things that weigh heavy on your mind, so that you can connect to the love that is always there.

1. From a comfortable seated position, place your left hand on your heart and bend your right arm at your side, with your hand out, palm facing up.

2. Observe your natural breath and connect to the things in your life that fill your heart. It can be people, experiences, pets, or loving memories. As you reflect on positive, loving reflections, bring your attention to your left hand and keep connected to your heartbeat.

3. As you recognize anything that disconnects you from that love, such as fear, hurt, or doubt, acknowledge it and imagine it like an object in your right hand. Then, gracefully lift your right hand up and back, releasing this disconnection over your right shoulder and behind you, then bring your hand back down in front of you.

4. Continue this meditation for three to five minutes, letting your right hand release anything that disconnects you over your right shoulder. When complete, bring your right hand over your left hand, which is over your heart. Breathe and connect to your heartbeat.

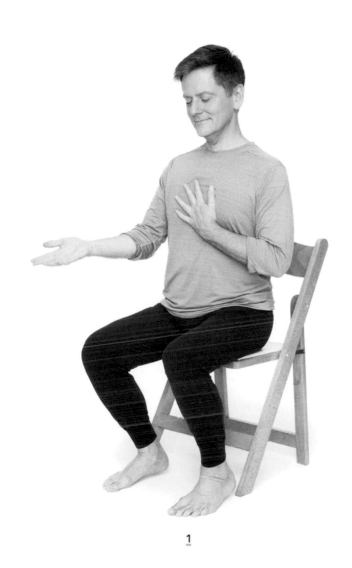

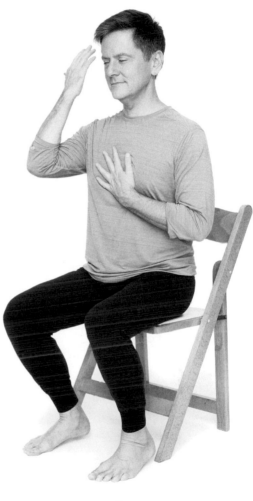

1

3

Flowing Gratitude

We have many teachers in our life, and grief is the unwanted teacher that helps us heal from loss. This is something we can be grateful for, since without it, we would not be honoring our loss at all. Our grief is a messenger that offers wisdom and guidance. Be with it. Thank your grief for what it has to share.

1. From a comfortable seated position, bring your palms together in prayer position at your heart.

2. As you inhale, sweep your arms up, and as you exhale, lower them down by your sides and bring them back together at your heart.

3. Repeat continuously, matching your breath with the motion of your arms, and as you flow, think or gently whisper, "Thank you." Allow the movements to embody grace and love and devotion to your loved one—for this is grief.

4. Continue at your own pace for two to five minutes. As you inhale, lift your hands up toward the sky and express gratitude, and as you exhale, sweep your hands down to your sides and back in front of your heart. When complete, release your hands to your side and breathe.

OFFER THANKS

During Flowing Gratitude, you can be both expansive and specific in what you say, such as: Thank you, grief, for healing my heart. Thank you, sadness, for allowing me to soften. Thank you to the divine for helping me experience this gift of life. Thank you for breaking my heart. Thank you for hearing me. Thank you for touching me. Thank you for loving me.

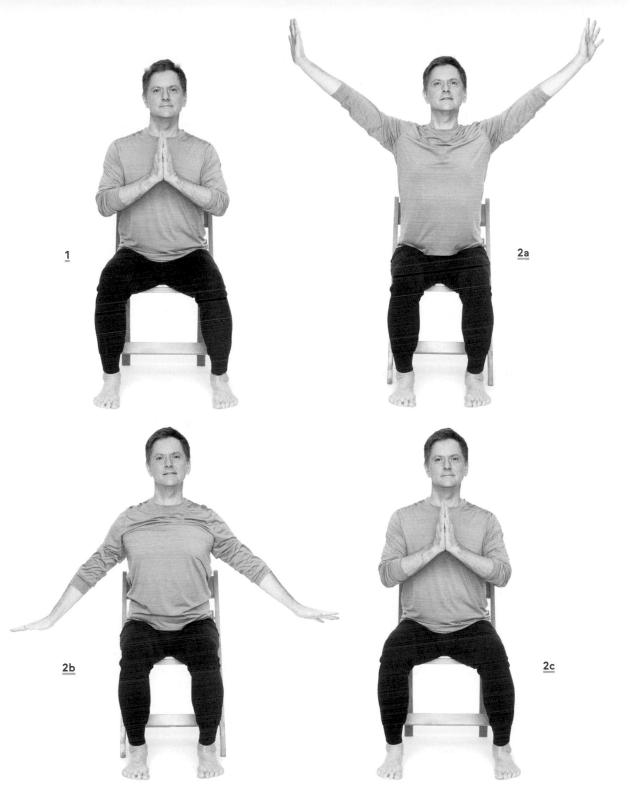

1   2a

2b   2c

Liquid Grace

We suppress so much pain in loss, and the hurt beneath the surface can be overwhelming. This moving meditation is a cleansing flow that helps connect you to spirit, to a power greater than yourself that will help you find kindness and grace as you wash away the pain.

1. From a comfortable seated position, release your hands down in front of you as if you're dipping your hands into holy water.

2. As you inhale, lift your hands up over your head, and as you exhale, flow your hands down, palms facing yourself and blessing your mind, heart, and body.

3. Repeat continuously, and as you move, think or speak this reflection: *I pour divine water to wash away the hurt. I wash away the feeling that I wasn't enough. I wash away the pain of not being loved the way I wanted. I wash away the embarrassment, shame, guilt, and humiliation. I bless myself with love. I wash myself in light. I am willing to forgive. I sit with the heartbreak and wash away years of unhealthy habits that no longer serve me. I wash away beating myself up. I wash away any obstacles that are preventing me from connecting with others. I wash away the anger or hurt that is still present. I cleanse myself and let it go.*

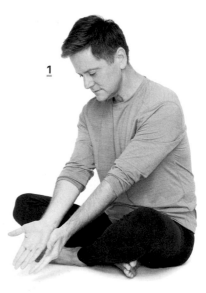

1

4. Continue at your own pace for three to five minutes. Keep flowing. As you inhale, dip your palms into a divine water of light and lift them over your head, and as you exhale, lower your palms as they bless your entire self—mind, heart, and body. When finished, come to a comfortable resting position and breathe.

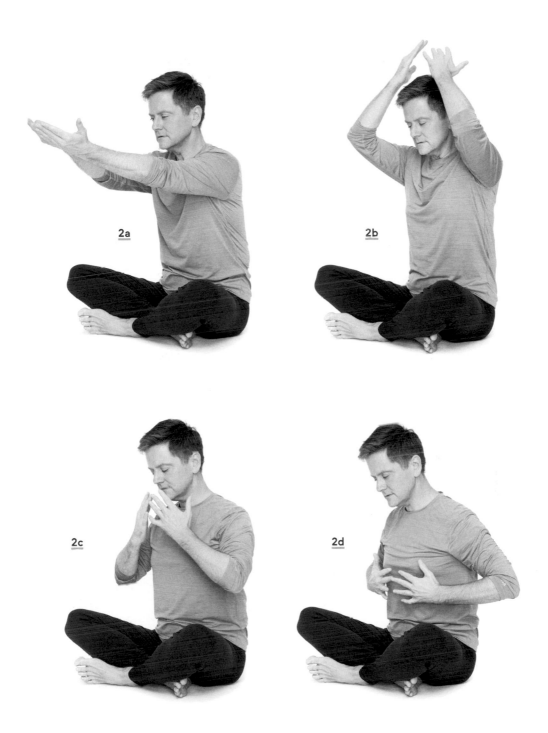

2a

2b

2c

2d

123

Appreciation Meditation

One of the fastest ways to shift our suffering is to connect to something we're grateful for, a connection that brings us deep love. This meditation helps quiet the mind so we can, for a moment, appreciate that love. This gives us a break from the pain and reminds us that there is goodness in the world.

1. From a comfortable seated position, place your hands out in front of you, palms up, with your left hand sitting gently in your right, and close your eyes.

2. Visualize a time, a moment, or a relationship in your life that you're thankful for. Try to see something specific; take your time to visualize this in detail in your mind's eye.

3. Next, say, "Yes," and bring your hands to your heart. Hold that moment gently and say, "Thank you."

4. When you're ready, place your empty hands out in front of you, palms up, and wait until another memory surfaces. Visualize this in your mind's eye, say, "Yes," bring your hands to your heart, and say, "Thank you."

5. Continue at your own pace for three to five minutes.

CONNECT TO SPIRIT

Appreciation can be for yourself, for another, or for spirit. Spirit can have many forms to many people: God, Jesus, Buddha, Higher Power, Universe. For me, spirit means love and light. That is our purest form. Allowing that light to flow through us is our highest form of honoring spirit. The law of nature teaches us that everything changes and fades away. We want to hold on to the things we love, but it's inevitable we will lose them. Nothing lasts. But we can appreciate what is and what has been.

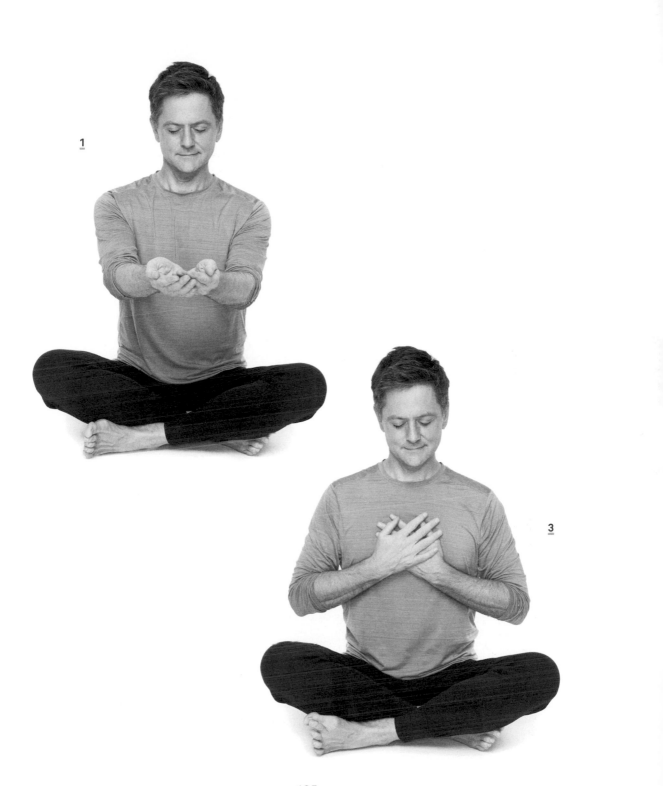

125

Extending Heart

It is normal to feel stuck, to feel unable to move forward with our grief. But there is so much to be grateful for, in our past, in our present, and in our future. This devotional movement of love is dedicated to those we are grateful for, those who have died, those who are with us now, and those who will support us as we move forward.

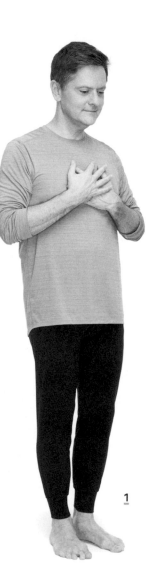

1. Stand with your feet hip-width apart with your hands at your chest. Lift one foot off the ground and then place it back down. Repeat with the other foot.

2. Continue walking gently in place, step by step, and connect to your breath. Then sweep one hand out to your side and bring your arm to your chest and hand to your heart. Do the same with the other hand, sweeping it out and back to your heart.

3. With this arm gesture, imagine gathering all that supports you and bringing it inward to your heart. Remind yourself of all the ways you are connected to those people you love and are grateful for, as well as to those who love and are grateful for you. Bring them close, sweeping in the love. Meanwhile, imagine stepping in place as a symbol of moving forward, while not forgetting the past. Even as you move forward, your loved ones will always be in your heart. You have lived and loved. You give and receive love today.

4. Continue walking in place and sweeping with your arms for two to five minutes. When finished, place your hand on your heart and become still. Connect and feel your gratitude and love.

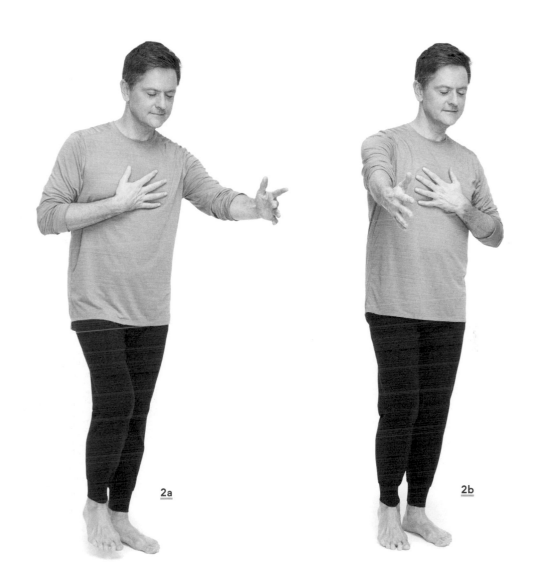

2a

2b

Heart Flow

———

This graceful meditation is a heart prayer that allows love to flow freely up and out, back and in, forward and out. As you flow this love forward and back, in and out, reflect on all the ways that love flows through your life, outward to others and back to yourself. Allow yourself to be loved by others; feel them loving you.

1. From a comfortable seated position, bring your hands to prayer position in front of your heart. As you inhale, lift your arms up, extending them to the sky, and whisper, "I love you." As you exhale, return your hands to your heart in prayer position and whisper, "Thank you."

2. On the next inhale, extend your arms forward and out from your heart, and whisper, "I love you." As you inhale, return your hands to your heart in prayer position and whisper, "Thank you."

3. Continue for three to five minutes, moving with this flow at your own pace and breath. Alternate extending your arms upward and outward, and feel your connection to that love. Don't grip it. Let it flow in its own divine way. Become an open vessel, allowing love to just flow through. When finished, center yourself in stillness and tune in to your breath.

LOVE IS ETERNAL

When a loved one dies, it may seem like the connection is gone. But their love for you is eternal. Endless. Unconditional. Their love is too strong to be knocked down by death. Their love still exists. Grief is love, and love is a connection that can never die.

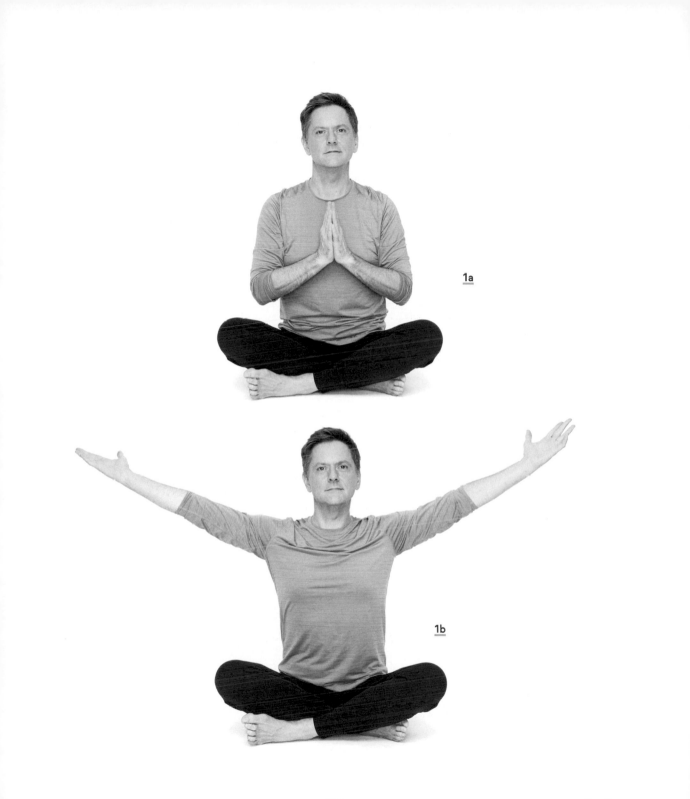

1a

1b

129

Continues

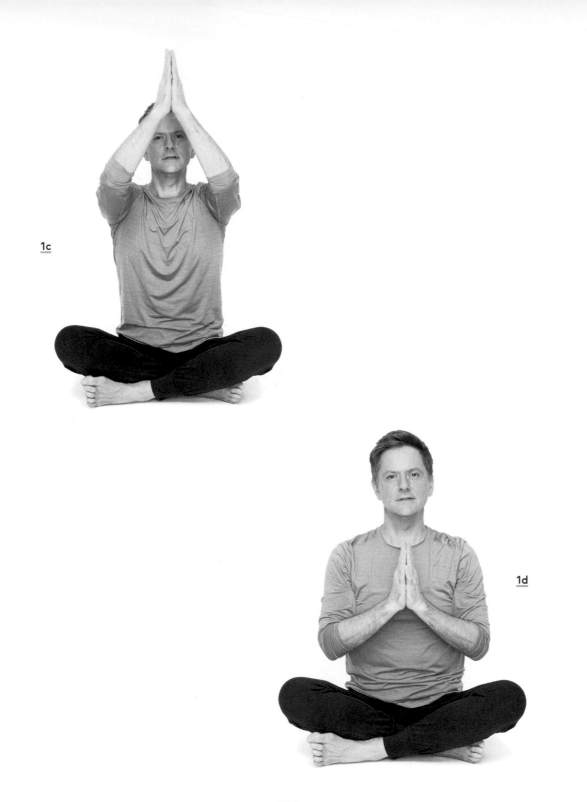

1c

1d

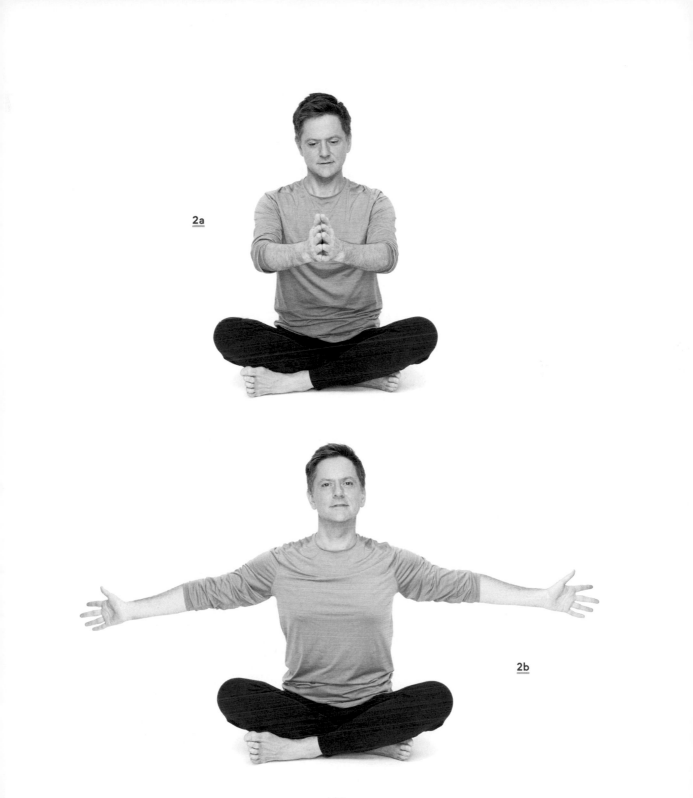

2a

2b

Loving-Kindness Meditation

———

Everyone wants loving-kindness and a sense of belonging. Are you willing to offer this to everyone, including yourself? Can you use this loving-kindness to connect to your loved one who is gone? We can wish to be happy ourselves, and we can wish it for them, too. As our love for them never dies, neither can our hope for their happiness, wherever they are.

1. From a standing position, with plenty of room in front of you, bring your hands to your heart.

2. Take one full step forward and reach your hands out in front of you. Extend loving-kindness outward and say, "May you be peaceful." Return your hands to your heart and say, "As I wish to be peaceful."

3. Take another full step forward and reach your hands out, while saying, "May you be free from suffering." Return your hands to your heart and say, "As I wish to be free from suffering."

4. Continue in this way, stepping forward, reaching your hands out, and voicing expressions of loving-kindness. Use your own phrases, or use the ones below, adjusting them so they feel right:

   - "May you be happy, as I wish to be happy."
   - "May you be free, as I wish to be free."
   - "I wish you love, as I wish myself love."
   - "I wish you peace, as I wish myself peace."

5. When finished, rest in a standing position, bring your hands to your heart, and offer yourself loving-kindness.

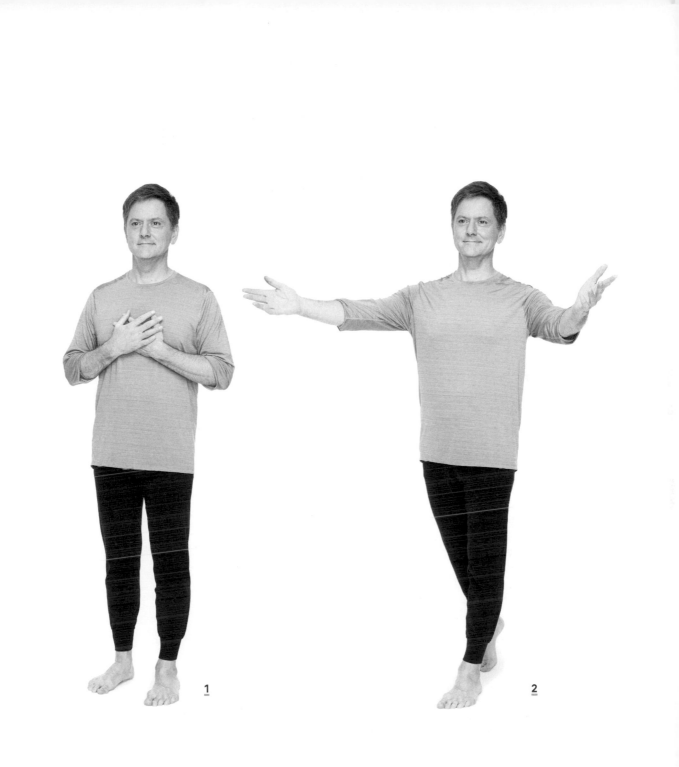

Om Mani Padme Hum
Meditation

———

The mantra *"Om mani padme hum"* is thousands of years old. It contains all the teachings of the Buddha—love, compassion, forgiveness, tolerance, and self-discipline. It transforms the root of suffering through sound, so that when you repeat it over and over, it brings us to a place where our suffering can be shifted into pure consciousness.

OM is the sound/vibration of the universe. It destroys attachment to the ego and establishes generosity.

MANI means jewel. It removes jealousy and desire as you find ethics and patience.

PADME means lotus. It represents moving from darkness into the light. It transforms prejudice and possessiveness into perseverance and concentration.

HUM represents union with spirit. It removes hatred and connects you to wisdom and purity.

This phrase helps to shift impure levels of thought to transform the root of suffering within our emotions and mind. By repeating this mantra, we cultivate enlightenment by creating an emptiness of the ego and of the belief of separateness.

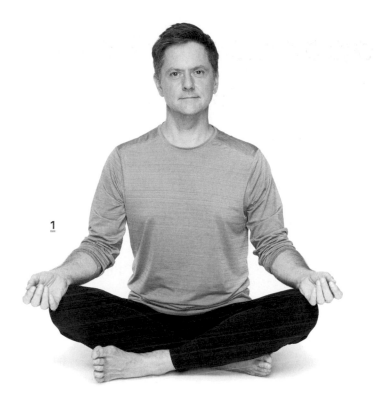

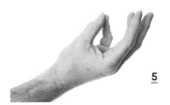

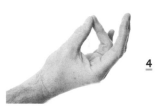

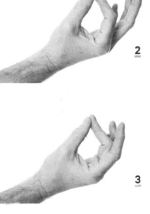

1. From a comfortable seated position, place your hands on your knees, palms up. Observe your natural breath, and then begin to recite *"Om mani padme hum"* out loud, touching the four fingers with your thumb with each sound.

2. **Om:** Touch the thumb to the index finger.

3. **Mani:** Touch the thumb to the middle finger.

4. **Padme:** Touch the thumb to the ring finger.

5. **Hum:** Touch the thumb to the pinky finger.

6. Continue this meditation at your own pace for five to seven minutes. When finished, come back to silence.

Ho'oponopono Flow

Forgiveness is a medicine that can help heal our soul. This practice is based on the ancient Hawaiian prayer known as Ho'oponopono (pronounced ho-oh-po-no-po-no), a word that means "to make right." This prayer brings balance to the self and to all relationships, even with our ancestors. It encourages taking responsibility for everything in our life. It is a powerful way of letting go of the most challenging life experiences.

1. From a comfortable seated position, lift your arms up from each side, with elbows bent and open palms facing the sky.

2. Inhale deeply, and as you exhale, turn your palms down, lift your elbows up, and round the spine as if you were opening the back door of your heart.

3. As you inhale, arch your chest forward, bring your elbows down, and turn your palms up, as if opening the front door of your heart.

4. Repeat this sequence so that it flows, alternating your arm position like wings, and arching and bending your spine. As you do, repeat out loud: "I am sorry. Please forgive me. Thank you. I love you."

5. Continue at your own pace for two to five minutes. Be open to what comes up for you. Acknowledge and allow the meditation to gracefully heal any hurt. All you need is willingness.

OPEN UP TO FORGIVENESS

In the ancient Hawaiian prayer Ho'oponopono, you connect to these four powerful phrases:

"I am sorry. Please forgive me. Thank you. I love you."

Whatever past grievance you're dealing with, by committing to this mantra, you become open and willing to release the hurt.

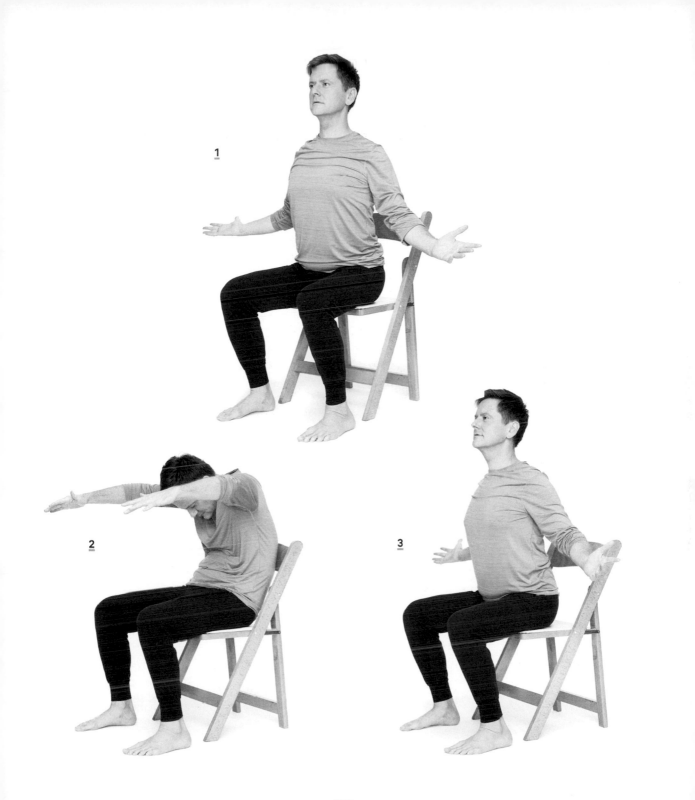

137

Circle of Life

The "circle of life" refers to how everything that is born also dies. Every flower, every plant, every person—whatever lives has an end. But the circle of life also reminds us of our wholeness, for just as a circle is complete and without end, so are we. We come into this world whole, we continue to live in it whole, and we leave it whole.

1. Stand with your feet hip-width apart. Bend your knees slightly with your hands at your sides. As you inhale, lift and stretch your right arm up, sweeping it toward the left side of your body and up and around your body. As you exhale, your arm descends and returns to your right side.

2. Make the same circular motion with your left arm. Inhale as you lift your left arm up, sweeping to the right and then over your head, and exhale as your arm descends and returns to your left side.

3. Next, as you inhale, bring your palms together in prayer position, then lift and raise your hands over your head, and as you exhale, spread your arms out, sweeping in both directions and returning them to your sides.

4. Repeat this sequence of three circular arm movements, and as you do, connect to a power greater than yourself. Move with grace. Honor your circle of life, your loved one's circle of life, and connect to Divine Spirit, allowing it to expand your circle. Feel your grief; allow it to flow. Even in grief, you are whole.

5. Continue at your own pace for three to seven minutes. When finished, relax your arms and come back to your natural breath.

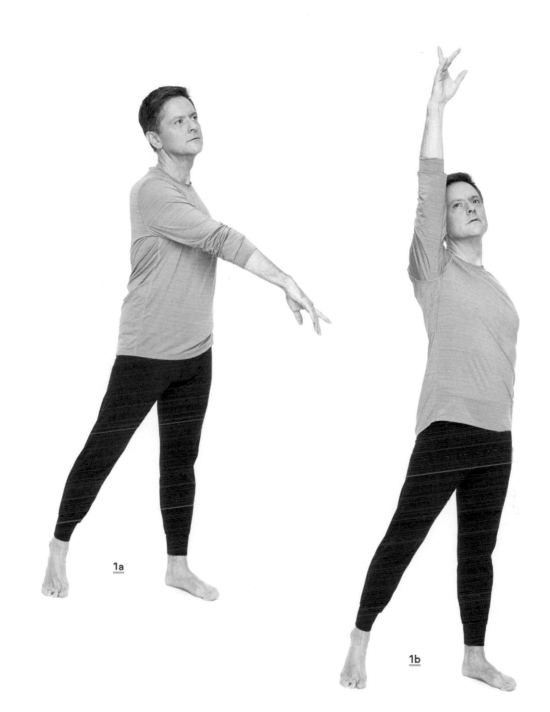

Continues

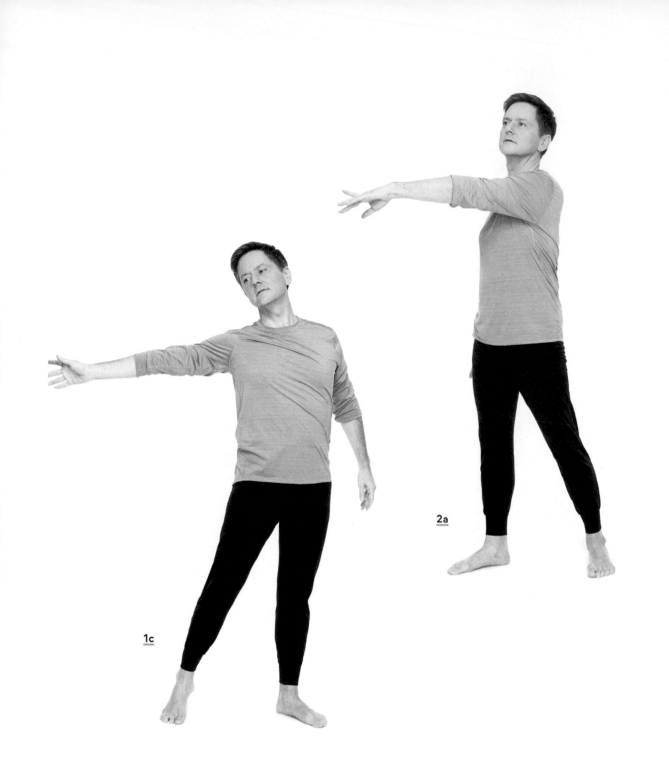

1c

2a

140

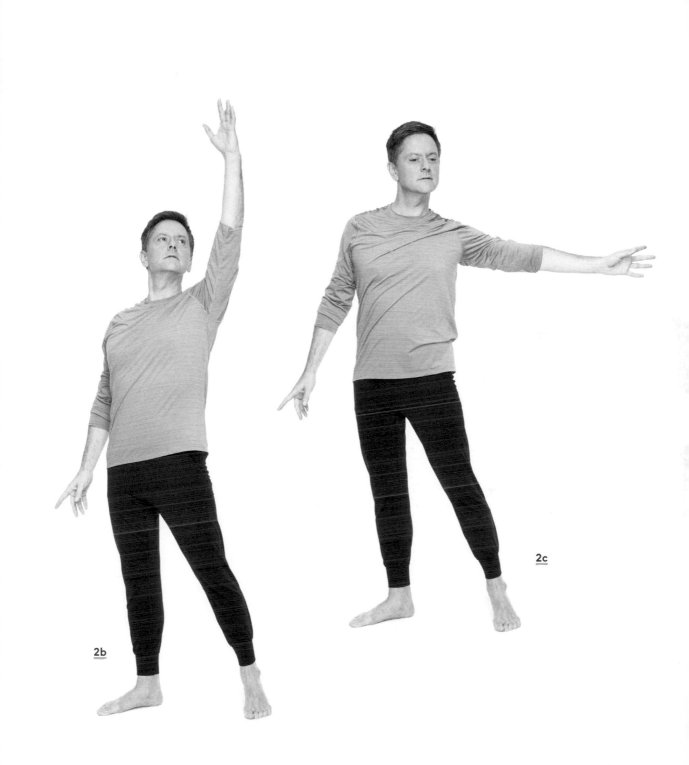

2b

2c

141

Continues

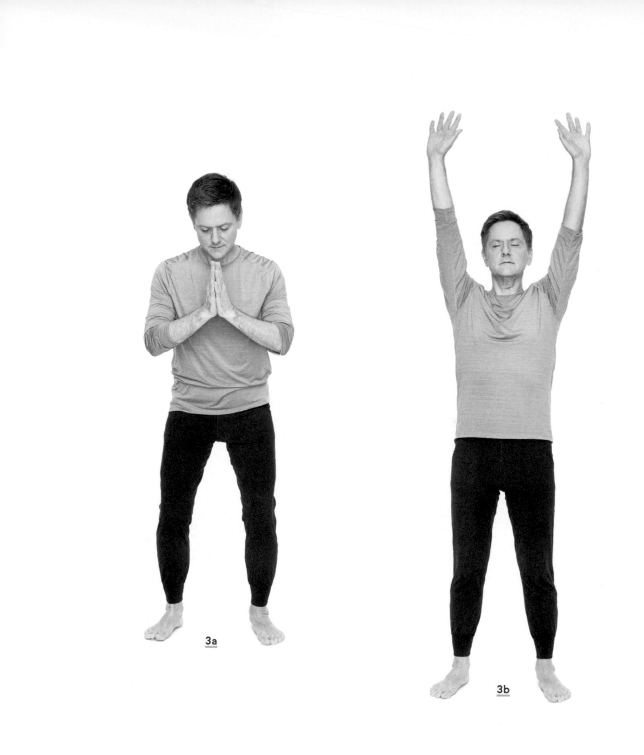

3a

3b

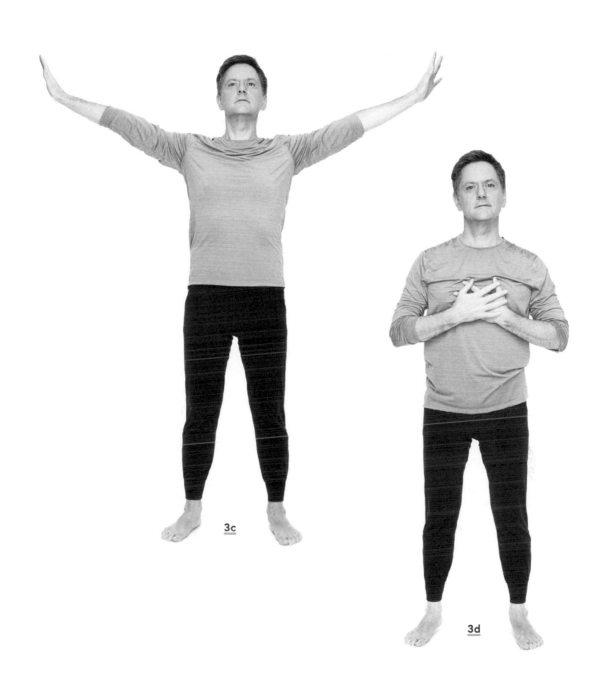

3c

3d

Dance Prayer

———

This beautiful expression of love allows your grief and love to flow. Dance Prayer is a sacred movement experience of Grief Yoga—it is body prayer that expresses itself in any way you choose. There is no way to get this wrong. This is simply an offering of the heart.

Before you begin, select a song to dance to, something that moves your heart and soul, that expresses what your heart wants to say, or that reminds you of your loved one. Some suggestions might be "Hallelujah" by k.d. lang or "The Prayer" by Andrea Bocelli and Céline Dion. Also, make sure you are in a clear space with room to move.

1. From a standing position, place your hands on your heart or bring your palms together in prayer position and breathe. Imagine your space filled with light. Invite into this space all of your ancestors, invisible supports, angels, spirit guides—all those you cry and sing and pray to. Offer your prayers, your longings, your thanks. If you want to dedicate this song to someone who has died, you can whisper their name before you begin.

2. Turn on your song and let your body move and dance to the music in whatever way it wants. Your eyes can be open or closed. If you don't move at all, that's okay. There is no way to do this wrong.

3. As you flow and breathe, allow this dance to be an offering. Let your prayer come from your heart and your soul. This is your time, your Dance Prayer. Let this dance be a direct line of communication to your beloved. All it requires is a willingness to be open. As you explore, ask yourself: *How can I open? Can I stay open?*

4. When the song ends, come to a comfortable seated position and let yourself be in stillness. Just breathe and acknowledge whatever occurred. Embrace whatever you're feeling.

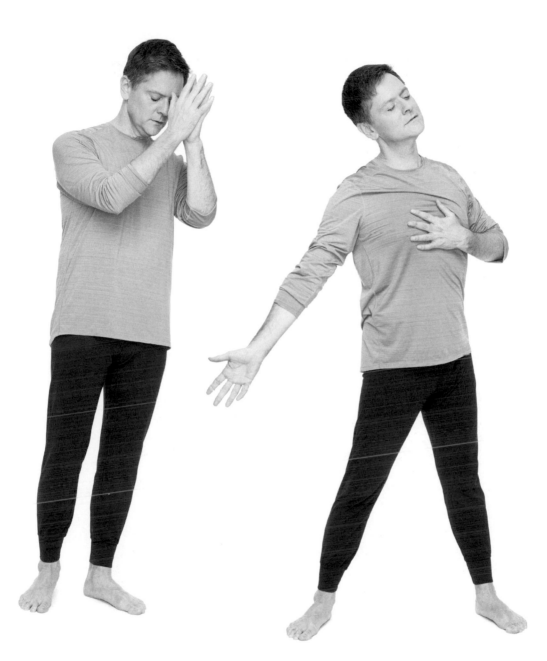

145

Continues

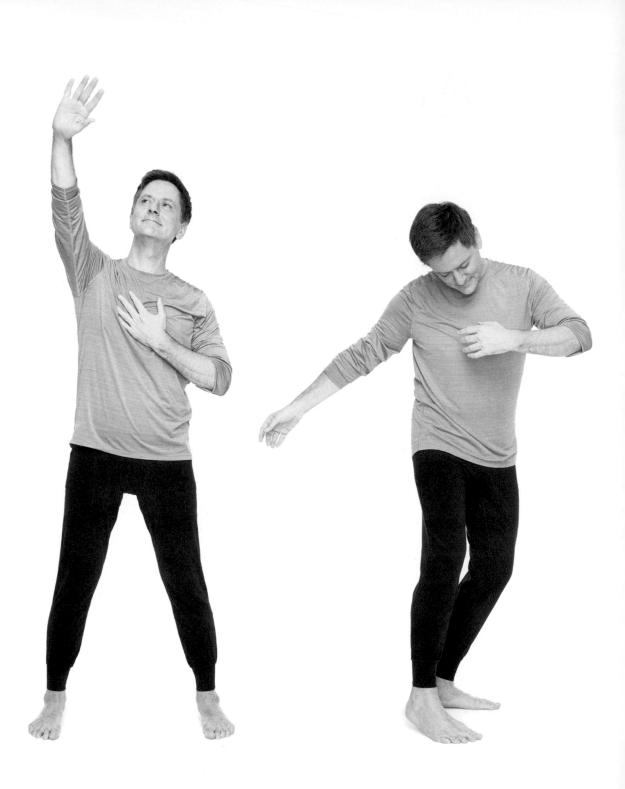

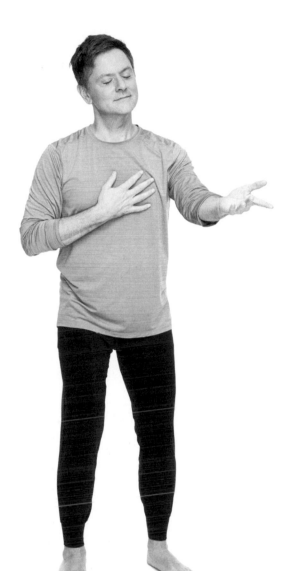

FEEL THEIR LOVE

When your Dance Prayer is finished, let everything be just as it is, with nothing to change. Be okay in your vulnerability, and consider whatever you discovered or witnessed. What qualities emerged in your Dance Prayer? Did you connect to your love? Close your eyes and feel your love for that person, and feel them spiritually loving you. Be open to feeling the presence of all your angels and guides. If you wish, say, "Thank you."

Moving into Surrender

These flowing meditations are meant to connect you to positive memories of loved ones and to compassion toward yourself.

The exercises in the step of surrender are meant to help you slow down, stretch, breathe, and soften your mind and body. Embrace these restorative practices by relaxing and letting go within. It's possible through letting go to stay present to love and lean into more peace.

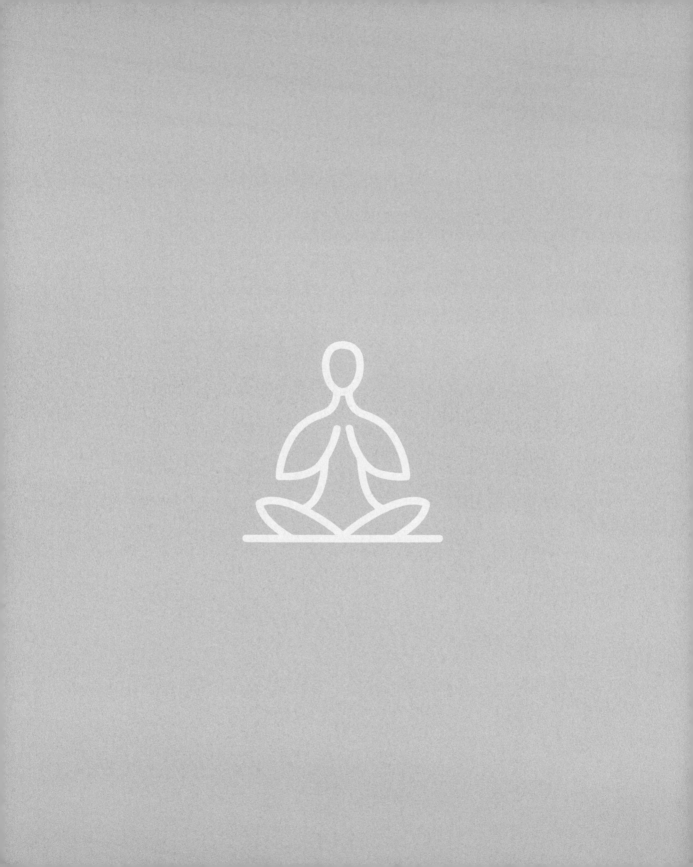

4

Surrender

We must be willing to let go of
the life we planned so as to have the life
that is waiting for us.

—JOSEPH CAMPBELL

Surrender guides you to accept what is and creates the space to restore. Be willing to soften your mind and body with compassion. Your love will guide you toward more peace.

Surrender is the practice of letting go. We surrender to something greater than ourselves. That can be God, Universe, the Divine Spirit, Creative Consciousness, or a Higher Power. We can surrender to love, to those who are living or dead, and we can surrender to self-love, which is often the most difficult but most important kind of love to embody. We can surrender to the strength and fire that lives within us, that helps us move through our grief. We can surrender to what we're feeling, whether it's sadness, anger, love, or joy. We can surrender to our emotions like a wave passing over and through us.

We all have to let go of things in life. Our job, our work, those dear to us, and our own physical bodies. Change is the only constant in this life. Loss is a change we don't want, and it happens despite our feelings. But if we are open and lean into what is, this letting go can guide us to a place of acceptance. Accepting reality for what it is. Accepting that we don't have to like a situation even as we recognize what is. It's normal to want to keep fighting, to resist letting go of those we hold dear to our hearts. We want to grasp tightly and not let go. Can we accept and surrender into hurt and pain and know that this too shall pass?

Surrender can be seen in a positive way. Instead of fighting something that can't be changed, we accept what is and stop fighting it. We surrender to the fact that there is a lot of work to do. When we trust, we can let go.

Some people perceive letting go as a sign of weakness, but there is a gift in surrender. There is a strength in making peace with reality.

I didn't want to let go of my sister, my dear friend, my dog. And yet there are times when life forces us to release, and we simply must let go. If you surrender to that inescapable letting go, you connect to the mystery of life. What is living, even

150

in this letting go? What happens when someone dies? It's a mystery. But there can be a peace in letting go and a curiosity about what's next.

Still, we can resist. How can we surrender someone we loved so deeply?

I begin by remembering that a part of the person still lives in me. Their memories remain. Their love still lives in my heart. And I allow the possibility that I can create something that honors both that love and that loss.

FINDING TRUST AGAIN

How can we develop trust when we're dealing with death? We know death exists and comes for all of us. No one ever lies about that. But to get through our days, we have to trust that death is *not* coming yet, not now or in this moment, or else we would live in constant fear.

Once death comes, how do we trust again? How do we trust the divine flow of life? How do we trust that there are angels in spirit and in human form that are here to guide us and take care of us? How do we trust in a power greater than ourselves, whether we call it Source, Earth, God, or Universe? How do we trust that love will continue to live in us?

> **In trust, there is an inner knowing that connects with faith.**

In trust, there is an inner knowing that connects with faith. It gave me the ability to surrender and let go of my sister, Ella, because I trust that we will be reunited in heaven. Death is not a betrayal. It is an ending we know must come eventually, the closing of a chapter, but the story continues. Our story continues, despite this death.

The act of surrendering brings us to a place of strength because we are connecting to something greater than ourselves.

What does surrender mean? When we surrender, we affirm: *I recognize that my loved one has died, but I can surrender to the possibility of their spiritual presence and the gift that it brings me.*

Surrender is about accepting love, no matter what is going on. It means that even in the midst of our greatest pain, we can believe that all things are possible. We can move toward peace and even happiness. When you move toward finding peace within, you quickly discover that you are exactly where you're meant to be, and everything is okay. As we move step by step in our lives, we remember that each step doesn't have to be perfect. We are a work in progress. You are a mighty person in the making.

Suffering is real. Death is real. Developing a relationship with death forces us to evaluate the life we've lived, to accept it and say, "I've done okay. I did the best I could."

This isn't easy, but it is the journey of our lives to get to a place of surrender. Embracing intuition is the path. Don't seek the answers outside of yourself. Instead, become still and connect to your own wisdom. There's no need to force it or even to try. Wisdom lives within all of us in each moment—the fire within, the grace and flow, the wind of constant change, the earth of deep foundation, the space and universe of expansion. Each of these helps us to see the unity within, connecting us to this world and to the universe.

When depression weighs heavy on your mind and soul—and it will, from time to time—it's important not to lose faith. Where does spirituality live in this dark moment? What helps you to lift your spirit? Whether it's prayer, nature, God, yoga, or meditation, lean into that. In your worst moments when nothing seems to help, say a small prayer: "Help me find my way. Help me."

FINDING SURRENDER

Shana's son, Jeffrey, died from an overdose, and she didn't know what to do. His death devastated her. She didn't know if she could keep moving forward.

When she attended a Grief Yoga class, I could see how her energy was depleted. She had been through the largest challenge she had ever endured, and she needed support.

I invited her to move into Sphinx pose (page 156). Shana laid on her stomach with her chest lifted and her elbows under her shoulders, as if opening the front gate of her heart. I asked her to silently say her son's name, Jeffrey, and be open to the love that is still present. The love that didn't die. After holding the pose for six to eight breaths, she came down to Wisdom pose (page 158), placing her hands underneath her forehead, palms down, and just breathed.

Tears were pouring down her face. "I just want Jeffrey back," she said. "I feel so lost without him. I want my life back." As she cried, I sat beside her and breathed with her.

She didn't need my advice. She didn't need me to respond. She just needed someone to witness her heartbreak, to sit beside her and let her know she wasn't alone.

As she rested in Wisdom pose, she said, "I know Jeffrey wants me to keep living. To keep experiencing life. I just need to find the motivation."

Eventually she moved onto her back and into Bridge pose (page 164), with her knees bent, her feet on the earth, and her hips lifted. This pose embodies a "bridge of healing." She felt she had lost her way, and this posture symbolically embodied her path forward, the path of remembering the love they shared. This path would guide her from devastation into hope for better days to come. Even though her heart was broken, she was open. Shana was doing her best to move forward, to open and breathe, and to surrender.

This isn't easy, but it is the journey of our lives to get to a place of surrender. Embracing intuition is the path.

We moved into a Knee Down Twist (page 178) to gently twist her spine; this posture embodies how life can twist and turn in unforeseeable ways. As much as we want to control things, many times we can't. Losing Jeffrey was a twist of life Shana couldn't control, but this physical twist was something she could manage. So was the balance of life.

At the end of class, when Shana lay in a resting pose called Savasana (page 182), I could see that her eyes were open. She couldn't quiet her mind. She didn't know how to find peace.

"Just come back to your breath," I said gently. "Just be willing to let go."

"I don't want to let go of Jeffrey. I don't want to let go of my son."

"Can you let go of the pain?"

"I don't think I can," she said.

And that's all right. We can surrender only to what we allow, and Shana wasn't ready to let go, not yet. Everyone heals at their own pace.

BROKEN AND BRUISED

Grief can knock us down, and after devastation, it's normal to feel broken.

Falling down is universal. We do it as children. It's how we learn to walk. What matters is how we get back up again. Do you beat yourself up for the fall?

One of my students took a big fall on her face and injured her neck. She was walking outside her home and tripped. Her eye was black and blue, her face was bruised, and she said she looked hideous. Gross. Horrible to look at. She couldn't stop crying. She didn't want to reach out to anyone. She felt ashamed of her fall.

Her physical wounds were bringing up emotional wounds. She said, "I'm such a failure. I've let so many people down. I just can't stop crying."

I reminded her that her tears were perfect. They were helping her heal her bruised eye, and they were helping her heal the wound in her heart, too.

A fall can be traumatic. It can stop us in our tracks. But when we surrender to the fall, we can ask ourselves—what's still working? What's getting stronger because of this fall? Perhaps it's our

Grief can knock us down, and after devastation, it's normal to feel broken.

resilience and strength. Perhaps it's our ability to learn how to ask for help from others as well as realizing how allowing others to help can be a gift we give to them.

Perhaps what's growing stronger is our acknowledgment of the fragility of life and of impermanence. We can be thankful for the little things that are still working, whether that's our sight, hearing, taste, hands, or heart. What is working? The truth is that our biggest falls can be our biggest lessons. Did the fall give us some wisdom? Perhaps our heartbreak can teach us not to take things for granted, to remember that tomorrow isn't promised.

There's a way to honor your hurt and keep moving. There's a way to take what is broken and put the pieces back together. When the heart is broken, it is open for the light to shine in.

As much as a bandage can protect a wound, so can air and water, so can kindness and love. There's an opportunity to create meaning from devastation. Like a phoenix rising above the ashes, new life can arise, but only if you surrender to it.

SURRENDER TECHNIQUES AND EXERCISES

Grief doesn't just bring us to our knees; it lays us flat out on the floor. It's unavoidable, and we must surrender to it in order to get up again. Just like after a fall, we must start where we are. We must orient ourselves, we must ground ourselves, and we must prepare for rising up again by stabilizing ourselves. By beginning to move again. The intention of surrender is to help you let go of the struggle in order to find peace. Explore the postures that feel right for you.

Sphinx

———

This posture is about surrendering to all the pain that has knocked you down, while keeping your chin up. You lift your head, knowing that you have the strength to live again. It is possible to surrender to pain while at the same time raising your head and heart to show your willingness to live, to honor those who have died, and to honor your life.

1. Lie down on your abdomen with your body prone along the mat. Lift your chest and hold it up by drawing your elbows directly under your shoulders, placing your forearms parallel in front of you.

2. Press your forearms and palms down, fingers flat and pointing forward. Relax your shoulders, drawing them away from your ears, and pull your shoulder blades back. Press your sternum and heart forward and lengthen your head up. Keep your lower back neutral and relaxed. Embody the posture of a sphinx.

3. Breathe and open the front gate of your heart. Visualize and connect to the ancient wisdom and love within. Breathe into your heart to find expansion and openness. As you do, open to the love that is always present. The love that never dies. Reflect on moments of giving and receiving love. Become aware of sensations of deep love and pain. Become aware that all your loving connections—from relationships past, present, and future—are present in your heart. Connect to hope for love in the future and for better days to come.

4. Continue for one to three minutes, or as long as you wish. Hold the pose and breathe into hope that all things will turn out for the best. When finished, lie back down and surrender.

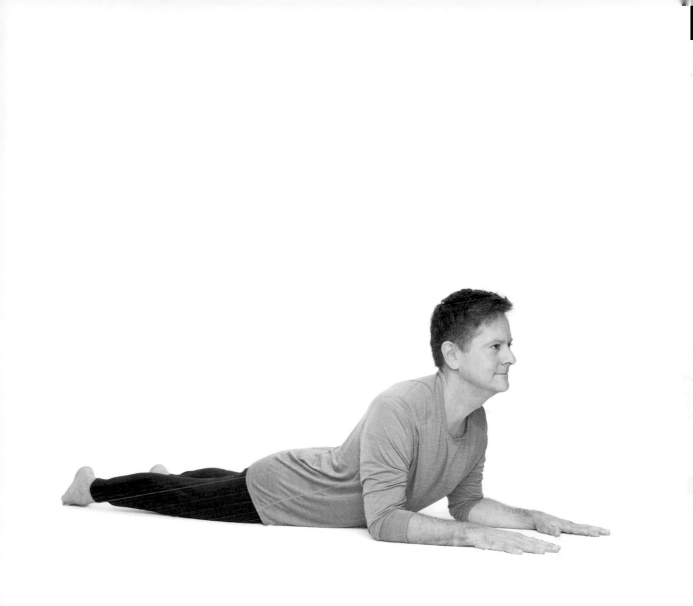

Wisdom

———

This deep resting posture helps to calm the nerves, opening you to wisdom while allowing the mind to rest. Grief brings the gift of wisdom, but it's an unwanted gift. We'd rather have our loved one back. This pose is about surrendering to the gift of wisdom that is available to us.

1. Lie down on your stomach on the mat, and place your hands under your head, palms down, one hand over the other. Rest your forehead on your hands for several breaths.

2. Move your hands to lie flat by your sides, and turn your head to one side, resting your cheek on the mat. Stretch your neck and hold for a few deep breaths.

3. Turn your head to gaze in the other direction, resting your other cheek on the mat. Stretch your neck and hold, taking a few deep breaths.

4. Return to the first position, bringing your hands under your head, and resting your forehead on your hands.

5. Hold and continue breathing deeply for one to three minutes, or as long as you wish.

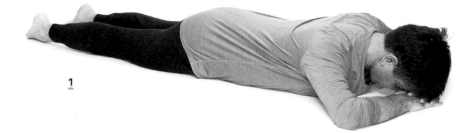
1

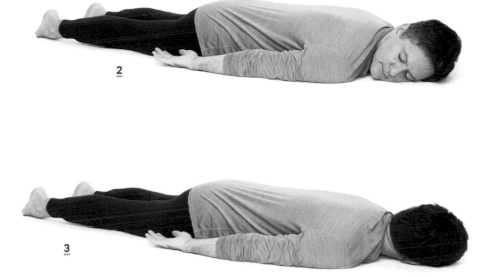

2

3

HELP ME TO SURRENDER

Surrender to the wisdom of what is. Surrender and bow down to the inevitable. When you feel resistance, all you have to do is say or think this soft prayer: *Please help me. Help me. I can't keep holding on to how I feel. I can't hold this burden alone.*

A soft prayer of help can provide a place for your vulnerability to shine through and your tender heart to exhale. A place where spirit can take over and guide you when your mind and body can't. Use any phrases that feel right, such as these:

Help me to forgive the resentments.
Help me to let go of this pain.
Help me to move forward from this depression.
Help guide me toward more light.
Help me to surrender.

Caterpillar

Just as a caterpillar has to climb into a cocoon in order to transform, this posture allows you to surrender into your transformation. Things have to be released in order for transformation to happen. The old reality has to be peeled away, and Caterpillar allows you to give in to that process, folding forward and surrendering what has been to allow what will be.

1. From a comfortable seated position on the mat, stretch your legs out straight in front of you, hands by your sides. Ground your sit bones down.

2. As you inhale, raise your hands above your head, lift your chest, and straighten your spine.

3. As you exhale, bend forward and reach for your ankles or toes, hinging from your hips. Drop your chin to your chest to stretch the ligaments at the base of your skull.

4. Fold forward as far as possible, placing your hands on your legs, ankles, or feet—whatever you can reach. It's okay to have a slight bend in your knees. Relax your leg muscles and spine as you breathe into this stretch.

5. Continue to hold this posture for two to four minutes. When finished, return to a comfortable seated position.

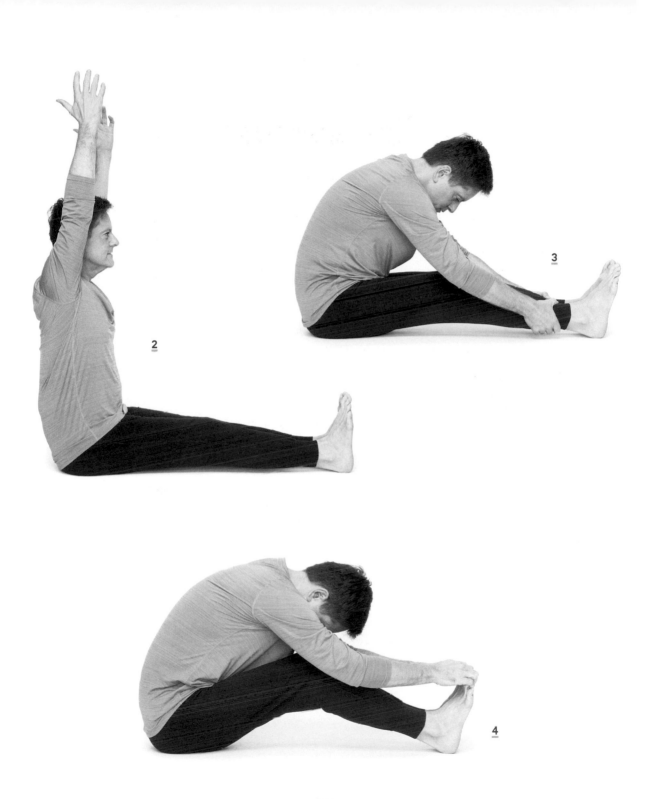

2

3

4

Butterfly

———

This grounded posture guides you to surrender and open your body as it calms your mind and helps you connect to spirit. It relaxes your lower back and hips and elongates your inner thigh muscles; as it does, allow your mind to relax and release old belief patterns. Surrender to the part of you that is eternal as you explore trust and patience.

1. Lie on your back on the mat, arms at your sides, and bend your knees. Place your feet on the floor, close together, and pull them in toward your bottom.

2. Let your knees fall open to either side, like the wings of a butterfly, so that the soles of your feet are together and facing.

3. Lengthen your spine and rest your head on the mat. If you wish, bring one hand to your belly and one hand to your heart. Embody surrender toward the earth and relax.

4. Continue for two to five minutes, simply holding the pose and breathing. Connect to healing energy as you visualize roots extending into the earth.

FIND TRUST

We all want change to happen quickly. We live in a quick society, and we want quick healing from grief. But there is no way to rush this process—grief is a state of being, not doing. Butterfly embodies the openness, the patience you have to find, that will allow you to quit doing and simply exist in the being of grief.

This can be frightening. You might wonder if it's safe to be in grief. Can you trust that you're going to be okay? To find trust in surrender, know that all your ancestors have experienced loss, too. Trust that your soul knows how to heal. Your soul knows how to grieve.

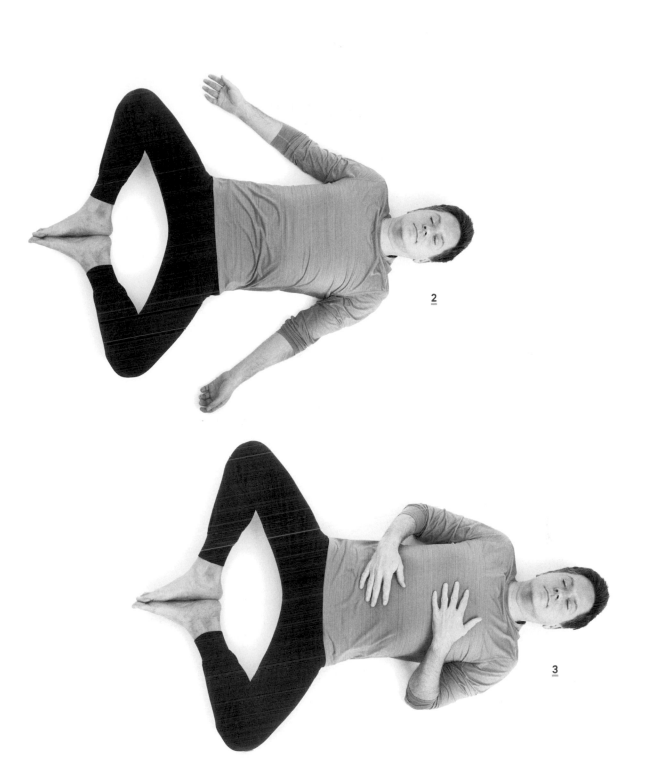

2

3

163

Bridge

———

When we swim in the troubled waters of grief, it can feel like we are drowning. Bridge allows you to recognize that you can rise above the pain, that you can surrender to it and allow it, but still remain in power, holding your heart high and open above the waters. You are more than just this pain, and you will live with more than just this pain.

1. Lie on your back on the mat, then lift and bend your knees, keeping your feet on the ground and hip-width apart. Place your arms flat by your sides, palms down, and pull your feet as close to your bottom as you can.

2. Pressing down with your arms for support, lift up your hips and then lift up your chest, making a "bridge" with your torso.

3. Relax your head and gaze upward, toward the sky. Press evenly into your feet and activate your legs. Hold this position for as long as you can.

4. When finished, lower your back slowly, rolling down one vertebra at a time, and lower your legs, hands at your sides, and breathe deeply.

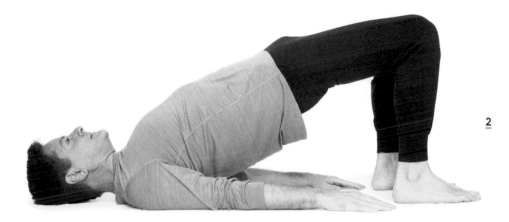

2

VARIATION

If you wish and it's comfortable, you can interlace your fingers under your back for a bigger opening of the heart.

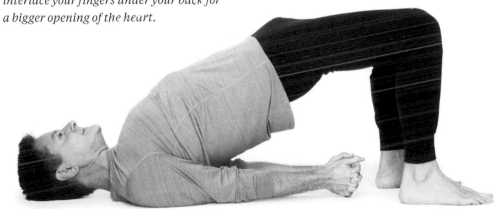

Pigeon

When we don't know what to do with challenging emotions, they often get locked into our hips. Tight hips can represent shame or fear of love, as well as emotional and physical trauma. The key is to breathe deeply and surrender into any discomfort. Use your breath to stretch, open, and let go, and be present to what is beneath the surface. Surrender to what is.

If you find this position difficult, try the Figure Four Stretch (next), which also opens and releases the hips.

1. Assume a tabletop position on your hands and knees. Bring your right knee near your right hand and relax your right hip to the floor. Adjust your right shin so that, as much as possible, it's parallel to the front edge of the mat.

2. Straighten your left leg to the back, so that both legs form a seven. Adjust your right hip back and your left hip forward. Support yourself with your hands, fingers spread wide on the floor, or bring your forearms onto the mat and rest your head forward and down over the right leg. Hold this position and breathe for one to three minutes.

3. Return to tabletop position on your hands and knees. Repeat this same position on the other side. Bring your left knee forward, relax your left hip to the floor, adjust your left shin parallel to the mat edge, and straighten your right leg back.

1

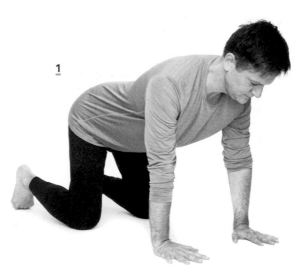

4. Hold this posture and breathe for one to three minutes. When finished, return to tabletop position and relax.

166

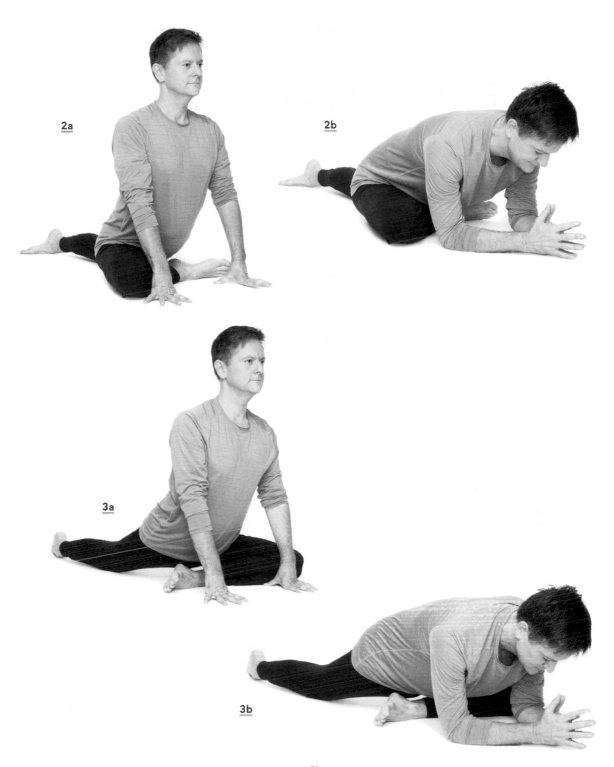

2a

2b

3a

3b

Figure Four Stretch

———

We are a part of the earth and the universe, a part of something much bigger than ourselves. As you lie on your back, picture the expanse of the sky above you. Surrender to that with humility.

1. Lay on your back on the mat, arms at your sides, and bend your knees, keeping your feet on the floor and hip-width apart.

2. Place your right foot over your left knee with your right foot flexed.

3. Interlace your hands behind your left thigh and gently, slowly, draw your left leg closer to your body. Hold and breathe into your right hip flexor and thigh for one to two minutes.

4. When you're ready, release your legs and return to neutral position, with knees bent and both feet on the floor.

5. Repeat the stretch on the other side. Place your left foot over your right knee, interlace your hands behind your right leg, and gently hug your right leg toward your chest. Hold and breathe into your left hip flexor and thigh for one to two minutes.

6. When you're ready, release your legs, stretch them out flat on the mat, and relax.

1

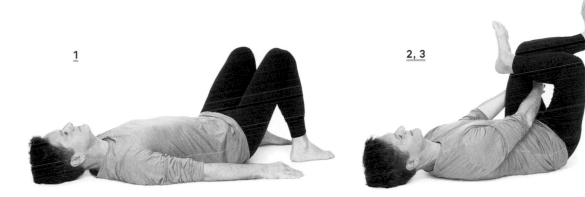

2, 3

4

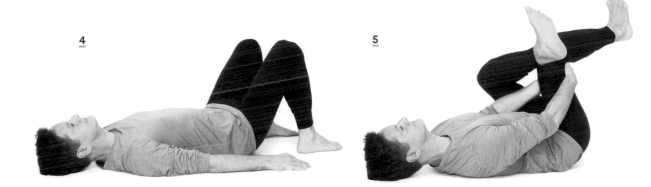

5

Half Tortoise

———

This relaxing posture stretches your back, shoulders, neck, legs, and hips to calm your heartbeat and improve blood flow to the brain; this can help with sleepless nights. Surrender connects us to the power of what is possible. When you surrender to what is, you give yourself over to the great unknown. This kind of letting go can help you find peace. Be open to what's next. Remember, when one door closes, another one opens.

1. Assume a tabletop position on your hands and knees. Bring your knees and heels together, and sit back on your heels, hands at your sides.

2. As you inhale, reach your arms up overhead, bringing your palms together in prayer position with your thumbs crossed.

3. As you exhale, slowly bend forward in a straight line from your tailbone to your fingertips. Stretch forward until your forehead rests on the ground and your hands, in prayer, rest on the earth. If your tailbone lifts up as you bring your forehead down, that's okay. Adjust to what your body needs.

VARIATION

If this position is too much for your knees, hips, or ankles, widen your knees out and adopt Child's Pose (page 54) instead.

4. Hold and breathe for one to two minutes, or for as long as you want.

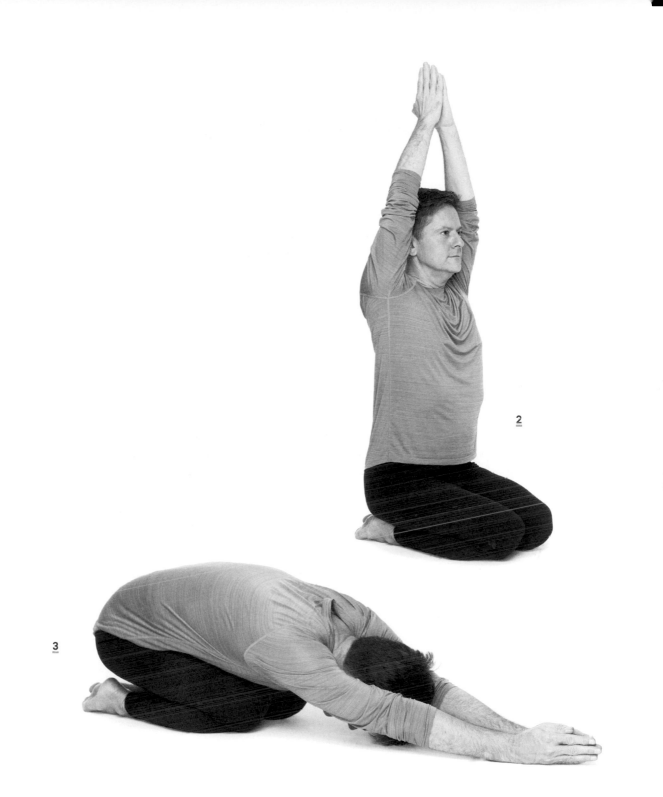

2

3

171

Legs Up the Wall

This relaxing posture helps to calm your mind into a meditative state. By reversing the effects of gravity, this posture helps to drain tension from your legs, feet, and hips, moving any fluids that build up from poor circulation or by spending a lot of time on your feet. As you let go, it feels like you're giving up, but in truth, you're receiving.

1. Lie on your back on the mat with your bottom against a wall, getting your sit bones as close as possible.

2. Extend and stretch your legs up the wall so the backs of your legs are resting fully against it.

3. Keep your arms slightly out to your sides and breathe deeply. If you wish or it's more comfortable, place a folded blanket under your hips to elevate them.

4. Hold this posture for three to eight minutes, then release and relax.

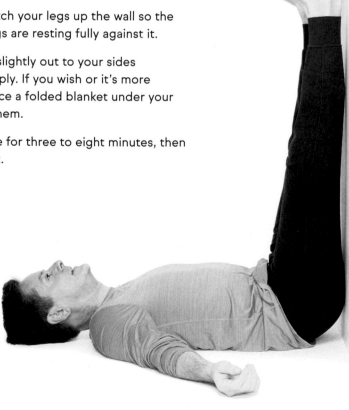

Fetal Position

Our life begins in this pose, and it's where we go for safety. It allows us to surrender into our origins—the place where we will end up. It helps relax your mind and body and creates a sense of security to find restoration. The healing powers of grief can transform a devastated life. Even in the face of death, new life can begin.

1. Lie on your back on the mat. Hug your knees to your chest and gently, slowly, roll onto your favorite side into a cradle position. Keep your knees bent with your heels toward your hips. If it's more comfortable, rest your head on your lower arm, while your upper arm remains around your legs.

2. Close your eyes and breathe. Hold this pose for as long as you want. Pregnant women should practice Fetal Position on the left side only.

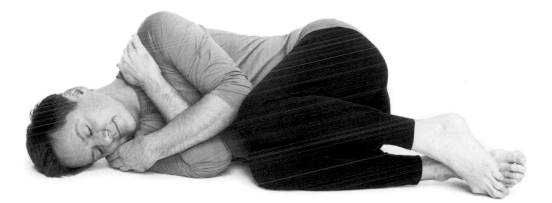

Frog

The hips are among the largest joints in our bodies. At these points, energy—such as anger, anxiety, and tension—can get stored. This squatting posture will stretch, strengthen, and relax your lower back, aid in digestion, and eliminate waste for healthy bowel movements. Opening the hip flexors will help with both physical and emotional constipation.

If this posture is too difficult for your lower back or if you experience knee pain, try Frog on the Wall (next), which is a restorative approach to this hip opening.

1. From a standing position, place your feet wide, heels in, and toes pointing out.

2. Lower your hips into a squat and bring your palms together in prayer position at your heart. If your heels lift a little off the floor, find grounding, balance, and support within the top parts of your feet.

3. Keep your knees in line with your toes, and gently press your elbows against the inside of your knees to open your hips farther.

4. Hold this posture for two to five minutes. If you need more support, place your back against a wall.

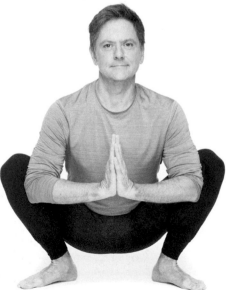

Frog on the Wall

———

Grief can leave us feeling depleted and questioning how to go on. This grounded posture allows you to surrender to what is without having to *do* anything. Sometimes it's okay to stop doing and just be. There is relief in simply sitting, listening, and finding stillness. Allow gravity to be your ally as you stretch your tired leg muscles, groin, and hamstrings.

1. Lie on your back on the mat with your bottom against a wall. Get your sit bones as close as possible and extend your legs up the wall.

2. Slide both feet down the wall and bend your knees, letting your knees fall open as wide as is comfortable.

3. Put your hands on your shins or knees and walk your feet out to the sides so that your feet are the same width as your knees. The wider your pose, the deeper your stretch, but move slowly and carefully, listening to your body. Don't force or push this stretch.

4. Hold this posture for two to five minutes, then release and relax.

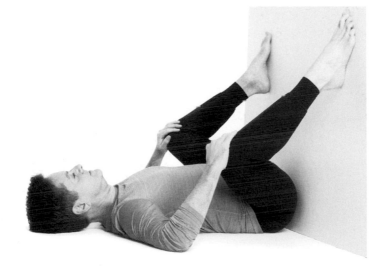

Knee to Chest

———

In surrender, we can do perhaps our deepest and most profound work yet—the work that's not about accomplishing and doing, but about being. We can connect to the eternal part of us that is just love. This stretch massages and purifies your abdominal organs. By stabilizing your pelvis and lower back against the earth, it helps ease lower back pain, allowing you to rest.

1. Lie on your back on the mat, arms at your sides. Relax your shoulders and pelvis, feeling them sink into the floor.

2. Bend your right knee and draw it toward your chest and shoulder, interlacing your fingers just below your knee.

3. Hold this posture for one minute. Breathe and keep your lower back and pelvis connected to the earth.

4. Release your right leg and return to a neutral position. Then repeat on the other side.

5. Bend your left knee to your chest, interlace your fingers below your knee, and hold this posture for one minute. When finished, release and relax.

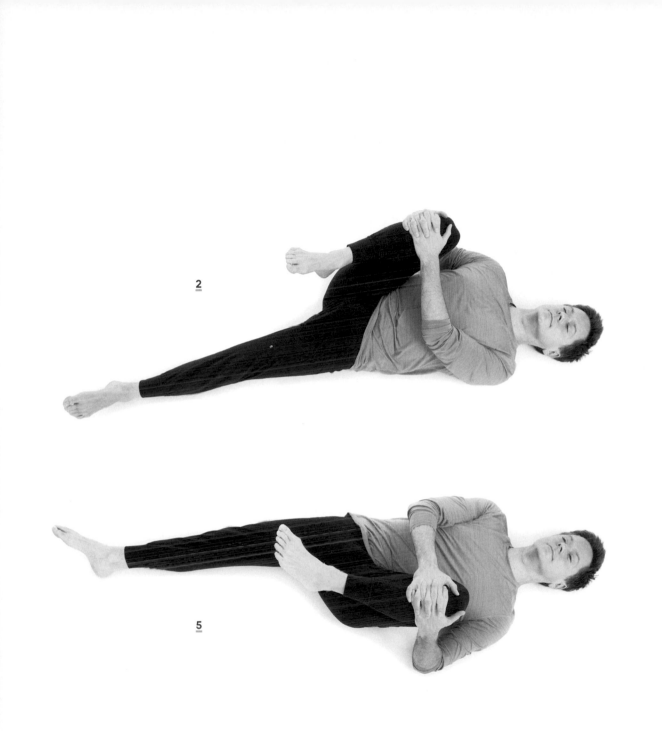

2

5

177

Knee Down Twist

———

Grief and loss can give us unexpected turns in life. This spinal twist allows you to guide the twist that's happening in your life at your own speed and pace. You can embrace this life and twist in your own way toward transformation. As you stretch, imagine that one side of you is the past, and the other is the future. You will embody both as you move forward, balancing the two.

1. Lie on your back on the mat, arms at your sides. Lift and hug both knees to your chest and give your lower back a massage on the earth.

2. Release your knees and allow them to fall to the left while extending your right arm straight out to the right at shoulder level. Let both knees and arm rest on the earth. As you inhale, lengthen your spine, and as you exhale, gently twist your spine farther. Hold and breathe for one minute.

> ### LET GO
> During the Knee Down Twist, focus on release and surrender, repeating to yourself the following statements:
> *I let go of the pain from the past.*
> *I let go of the former version of who I was.*
> *I let go of the tension.*
> *All I have to do is be.*
> *I'm going to be okay.*

3. Bring your knees back to center and hug them to your chest; align your lower back on the earth.

4. Release your knees and allow them to fall to the right while extending your left arm at shoulder level. Inhale as you lengthen, and exhale as you twist your spine. Hold for a minute, stretch, and breathe.

5. Come back to center, hug your knees to your chest, and rock from side to side, giving your lower back a massage. When finished, release your legs to the earth and relax.

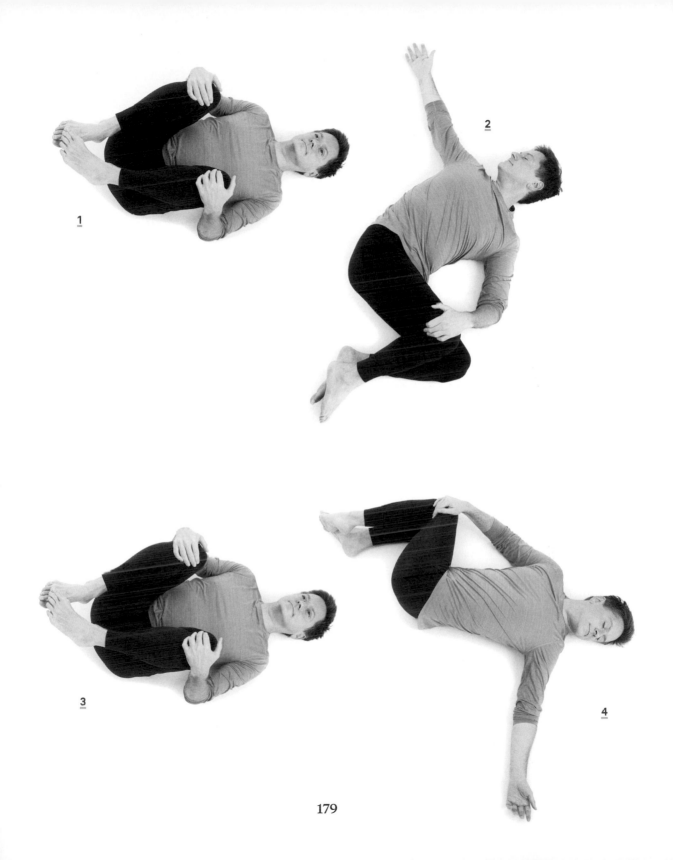

Happy Baby

———

This posture allows your spine to lengthen and your lower back to receive a massage from the earth. It calms your nervous system and creates length in your hips, thighs, and hamstrings. It releases tension in your lower back while decreasing your heart rate. Allow this grounding posture to help you tap into a place of innocence.

1. Lie on your back on the mat and bring your knees to your chest. Open your knees and grab the soles of your feet, ankles, or big toes, lifting your feet up to the sky.

2. Gently pull your knees down toward the floor. Feel the length of your spine grounded to the earth, from your tailbone up to the crown of your head. Allow your neck and shoulders to be relaxed.

3. Hold this position and breathe into your hips for one to three minutes. When you're ready, release your legs, surrender down to the ground, and breathe.

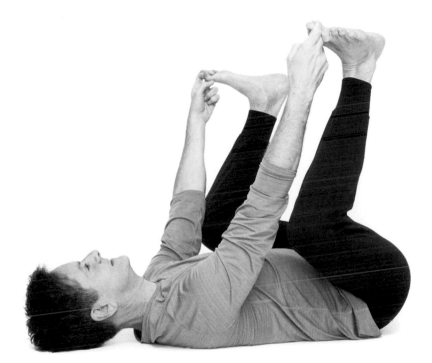

RECEIVE PEACE

This posture helps you surrender to a place of innocence as you slowly let go. You can surrender to what used to be, to what your life was like before your grief. This release can allow a deep blessing to emerge, one that lies beneath the surface. Receive it. Receive peace and harmony. Listen to the real you, the person who is funny, happy, and full of joy. You are still there.

Savasana

———

At the end of your practice, Savasana is a restorative posture that embraces a deep stillness and rest. Let your thoughts, emotions, breath, and body sensations merge into an experience of oneness with all that supports and surrounds you. Allow compassion, love, and openness to fill your body and mind. Let love inspire you. Let love connect you to what is divine, tender, patient, and forgiving.

1. Lie on your back on the mat, arms at your sides and palms up, legs flat and straight, with feet about hip-width apart. Relax your legs, shoulders, arms, and head. Allow your whole body to surrender to gravity. Let your feet fall naturally out to the sides. Relax the muscles in your face.

2. Close your eyes and observe your natural breath. Continue to relax your entire physical body and breathe. Sense your body coming into stillness and your muscles releasing into your bones.

3. Continue in this posture for as long as you want, whether for three or thirty minutes. Rest and surrender, just be.

REST IN PEACE

By lying on your back and letting go, you surrender to a place of deep stillness and being. As you surrender your body, you can bring your mind to your loved one who has died. Picture your loved one's face, imagining them at a happy time in their life. See their eyes sparkle. Feel the connection between the two of you that continues even now. In grief, it's easy to believe that your love left with that person and you are now empty. In truth, that love is still in you. The person lives in your heart. Wish peace for yourself as you wish for your loved one to rest in peace. Believe one day you will see each other again. Surrender completely to your higher self.

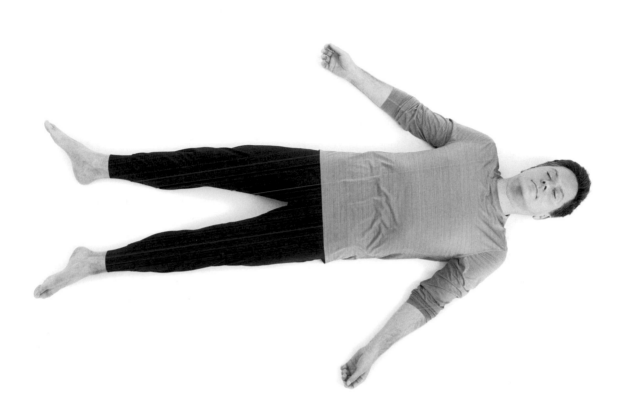

These restorative surrender techniques soften your mind and body. You recognize you're not the same person after this heartbreak and trauma. Amidst the loss, you can awaken to new possibilities. You can stand back up and move through the pieces of your life that are broken or overwhelming and tap into a deeper resilience, maybe even learn to laugh again.

You have a choice in how you move off your mat and into the world. The step of evolution explores ways to move forward in life to transform loss into empowerment.

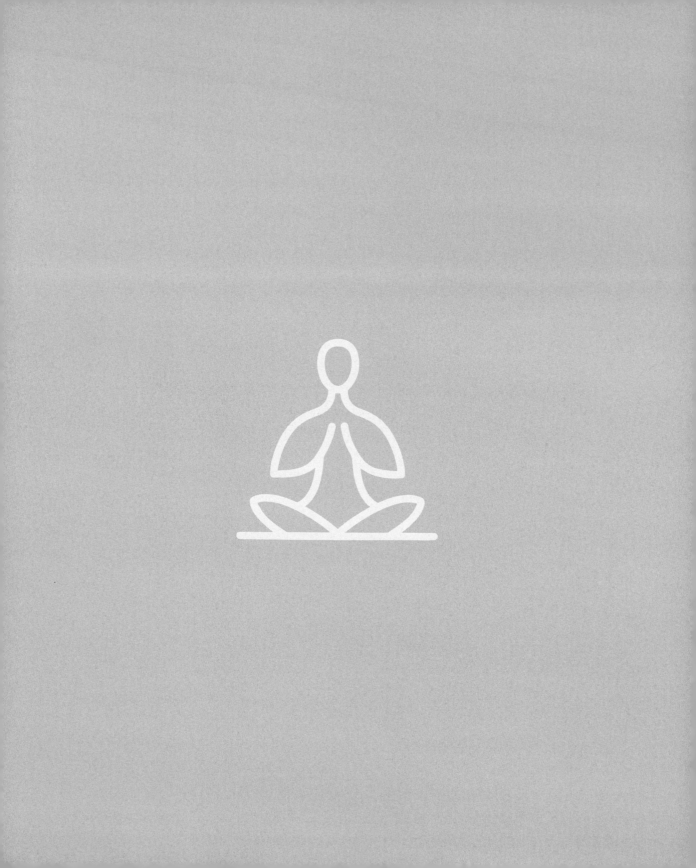

5

Evolution

You will heal and you will rebuild yourself around the loss you have suffered. You will be whole again, but you will never be the same. Nor should you be the same, nor would you want to.

—ELISABETH KÜBLER-ROSS AND DAVID KESSLER

Evolution guides us forward. When one chapter ends, another one begins. This loss can help you to grow and expand in ways you may not have realized. Let's move through the devastation toward more courage, balance, happiness, and empowerment.

If we love in our life, grief will be a part of our experience. The memories we shared with our loved one will always be with us. Grieving a loss may feel like the end, but in truth, we are moving toward a new chapter. We honor our loved one by living a life of happiness and purpose.

When you stand up and get off your mat, start moving. Remember that you are still alive. You can make your life beautiful. In this way, you can transform one step at a time. What will you do today to affect your tomorrow? Will you meditate? Do yoga? Create something in honor of your loss? Imagine a life of peace and purpose. When you are facing struggles, try not to get caught up in the drama. Listen to your body. What is it telling you? Don't run away. Investigate and see how precious life can be. Remember that you are a work in progress. You don't have to be perfect. Be present and okay with where you are in your pain, in your grief, and in your healing. The quickest way to complicate grief is thinking we are doing it too fast or too slow.

Evolution is the final piece of the puzzle in the cycle of compassionate transformation of Grief Yoga. It helps you accept and make the best of what is. Energy will flow wherever you place your attention.

Evolution does not mean letting go of grief. But in this final spoke in the cycle of Grief Yoga, we ask ourselves to grow and change, despite that loss. The paths to explore as we evolve forward are perseverance, purpose, and balance—all of which require hope.

Evolution does not mean letting go of grief.

CULTIVATING PERSEVERANCE

Even when we are suffering, we can choose how to respond to that suffering. After a death, we have to develop new skills for moving forward and adjusting to this new normal. We ask: *Who am I now after this death? How am I different after loving this person?*

One of the ways to shift suffering and change our attitude toward it is to embrace uncertainty and struggle and be open to learning. We can find expression and explore meaning in many different ways: through creating something that honors our love and the person, or by having an experience or remembering an experience that was meaningful.

This is an invitation to go on living, to make the decision to persevere and try. Our body is doing that anyway. Life is continuing. Our hair still grows, as do our fingernails and toenails. Our heart still beats, our lungs breathe. The truth is, each day we are moving closer to our own death. If we embrace our mortality and examine death, it's possible to be less afraid of it. How do you want to live in the face of death, knowing that death is coming? How can that concept help you focus on the life you still have? We are all slowly dying. We will die one day, but what about all the life we live until then? We're alive until we die. And the truth is, our worst fear isn't death—it's realizing we wasted the life we had when the time of death arrives. So the question becomes, how do we live?

Don't bury yourself before you die. Stand upright. Find meaning again, and care about your life and the love you feel. One way to do this is to live from meaningful moment to meaningful moment. Start now and embrace this moment, right here.

Enjoy what you have because life is finite. Make the choice to focus less on pain, struggle, and what you don't have, and focus more on love and enjoying what you do have.

DISCOVERING PURPOSE

If we don't transcend our struggle, it can feel like we aren't really living at all. But we can find purpose, even in the face of our pain. There are many ways to find purpose in life. We can begin by creating something from the heart. Or even a simple action or deed of love and service to another without expecting anything in return, as we transform our suffering and transition into service.

Purpose can be found by embracing the art in life and the beauty of nature, by savoring the pleasure of food and the caress and touch of love. It can be found by choosing not to rush through life but to embrace this moment.

Experience your life, and then ask yourself, what is the legacy you want to leave behind? Can you take the biggest heartbreak in your life and use it as fuel to create something that honors your loved one? It is possible to take something you perceive as negative and use it to create something positive and meaningful.

I think of my sister, Ella. I am still processing her death and her life. One of the ways I cope is by teaching Grief Yoga to people at cancer support centers. I offer a space for people to release some of their pain, to help them connect to more love and grace. I have found that it helps both me and my students to process the grief we feel. It helps us create meaningful memories with our loved ones.

When I teach, I think, *This is for you, Ella. I offer this because of you*. This helps me find meaning in Ella's death, to believe her death has purpose, that it can help relieve the suffering of others.

I worked with a woman named Megan who said she had a lot of shame in her grief after her husband died. She told me that she couldn't look at him at the end of his life. When he was dying of cancer, on his final day, he said, "Megan, I'm dying today."

If we don't transcend our struggle, it can feel like we aren't really living at all.

She told me, "I couldn't look in his eyes."

I saw her pain, longing, and confusion. I told her, "We all do the best we can. Your husband was consumed by cancer. I'm sure he didn't look well. It must have been brutal to see." Allowing me to witness her grief and pain was important for Megan. She moved from holding it all inside to saying it out loud. That was her evolution.

PUTTING YOUR GRIEF INTO PRACTICE

Love and grief are a package deal. If you choose not to grieve, then you choose not to love. Life is a path with many detours. There will be moments when you get lost, when you struggle. You may come to a fork in the road and have to choose which way to go. Remember that there are some paths that elevate and lift us up, and there are others that can lead us into the depths of sorrow and loneliness.

One path that can help in times of struggle is to be useful to another person who may be in pain. This is called Karma Yoga, which means taking the philosophy of yoga and putting it into action out in the world. There are so many ways you can put this into practice. You can help a friend who may also be in grief. You can become involved in a community, being of service to those who are struggling in some way. You can join a charity and support the work they do.

The heart of Karma Yoga is to act from a selfless place. It's about helping others and giving to those in need without desire for personal reward as you evolve from personal struggle to a place of service.

A student of mine, Jody, felt she didn't have any purpose or energy to carry on after her husband died. He had been her life, and after his death she couldn't find the inspiration to move forward. Regrets weighed heavy on her heart as she wondered, "If I had done something differently, would my husband still be alive?" As I helped her to express and move through the doubts and regrets that were challenging her, she accepted that he was gone, but she wanted to create something meaningful as a reflection of their love. She decided she could evolve by creating a garden of hope in an area of her backyard that was full of weeds. She placed a picture of her beloved in the soil and then she planted seeds and flowers. Her roses reflected their love. Bright pink orchids helped her remember their trip to Yosemite. Yellow sunflowers reminded her of his smile and laugh. Jody shared with me how meaningful this garden was to her and how it resembled the many colors of their love. It was also a lesson in the law of impermanence. Things are born, they blossom, and they die. She said to me, "What can I water today that honors my love for my husband and my life?"

The setback over a loss can knock us down. But it can also create great meaning within our lives as we move toward a new chapter. Honor your loved one by living a life of happiness and purpose. Create something that honors them.

As we move forward after loss, remember that it's not about the destination. This path doesn't *lead* anywhere. The path *is* the destination. And on this journey, you can learn to embrace all sides of yourself—your mind, your body, and your spirit.

SEEKING LAUGHTER

It can often feel impossible to think about laughter when you're in pain. However, at my retreats with David, after we have helped people process their feelings, we do Laughter Yoga. This can be challenging for the newly bereaved. Someone will often leave during the laughter, and David will be waiting outside. They tell him, "I can't laugh anymore."

Maybe laughter feels wrong, disrespectful, or they just can't let themselves do it. David says he understands and invites them to just watch the others laugh. At that point, the person has heard about everyone else's loss in the room. By inviting people to do Laughter Yoga, I want them to know that laughter is still possible.

A shy student of mine, Claire, had never done yoga before and was a little nervous. She walked to the back corner and put down her mat. She watched the others around her but she seemed isolated.

A little over halfway through class, after we had expressed and moved through the pain, I introduced my Laughter Yoga exercises (pages 206–213). "Honor whatever you're feeling right now," I said, "but use laughter as a way to move things through and clear out stale air. Take a step toward hope that you can connect with happiness. Invite the inner child to come out and play."

I could feel Claire's hesitancy and discomfort.

"I know this can seem ridiculous," I said, "but try to go with it. If you're irritable or angry right now, use the anger and let it come out with a laugh."

During the next few laughter exercises, I watched Claire laughing angrily with everybody else. She seemed to be getting a kick out of it, as if I'd given her the opportunity to honor whatever she was feeling and allow her laughter to move it through. Soon, the angry laughter turned to joyful laughter. Claire giggled as if she were a little girl on the playground. Everyone's laughter became contagious and joyful, and then out of nowhere, Claire burst into tears.

Our body reacts automatically when we laugh, even if we're faking it. Endorphins, the feel-good hormones, get released from the brain. Laughter assists with deep breathing, too. In grief, our breath can become shallow. The secret to deep breathing is not in the inhalation but the exhalation. Laughing is a great way to exhale all the air. When I did my Laughter Yoga training, there were times I didn't feel like laughing. I was irritable and tired, but since the body can't tell if laughter is real or fake, I decided to "fake it until I could make it." I laughed with my anger and irritability. The laughter became contagious and shifted into joy. When I felt anticipatory grief and couldn't process it, I laughed about my sadness until the tears started falling. Whenever I do this, I always feel lighter afterward.

It's okay to fake it until you make it. In fact, I recommend it. Laughter Yoga can help you change your perception of a challenging situation while it brings lightness and happiness into your life.

It's okay to fake it until you make it. In fact, I recommend it.

ACHIEVING BALANCE

Grief can knock us to the ground. We can lose our balance. Part of healing, part of growing and evolving, is finding our balance again. It's important to maintain balance in life, even if it's just a reflection of a single day. The sun rises and sets, the moon rises and sets. We need to balance *being* and *doing*. We cannot evolve unless we have both. There will be times when we need to take action and times when we need to rest. You know best which you are most drawn to. Are you running out and doing and doing and doing, avoiding being alone with your grief, with your inward self? Or, conversely, are you shutting yourself off and avoiding living your own life and finding your purpose? We all lean in one direction or another from time to time, and it is the work of a lifetime, over the course of every single day, to find the balance between them.

One client, Sarah, had so many losses, one after another, that she just kept running. She spent all her energy trying to be active and busy to avoid her sadness. One day she hurt her back and was forced to stop and slow down. Her sadness came crashing down on her. That lower back injury reverberated down to her feet, making it difficult for her to walk. Since she was a person of action, she knew she needed to do something about it, and so she came to yoga.

Tree Pose (page 216) was particularly difficult for her. When she explored it, it hurt her foot to balance and hold up her entire body. She wobbled and fell. "Remember, life is a continual balancing act," I said. "This is something we all have to work on, all the time. For now, in this moment, balance your effort with kindness." I suggested that she modify the pose: Rather than placing her foot above her knee as you're "supposed to," she could keep one toe on the ground, helping her to find her balance.

Sarah felt she had to "get it right" exactly, the moment she started. But life doesn't work like that.

Grief can knock us to the ground. We can lose our balance.

Tree Pose is about finding out what works for *you*. That is how you find your balance. When Sarah allowed herself the space and kindness she needed, rather than experiencing pain, she was able to feel the support of the earth. When she found that support, she raised her arms and her leg. Now she could rise up.

If grief leads to stagnation, remember that the secret to balance is movement. Imagine living and moving with grief as if you're relearning to ride a bike. If you're standing still, you cannot find your balance on a bicycle; it's impossible. How can these two wheels ever stay upright? By moving forward. At first, that movement will be rickety, and you'll probably fall over more than once, but eventually you will be able to find and maintain your balance. As we move through grief, we find a new kind of balance. It's different. It's not the life you had before, but it *is* a life.

In fact, balance requires both movement *and* stillness. We need *both,* and all of us have varying degrees of difficulty with them at varying times in our life. In yoga, we use the phrase "finding your edge." It means pushing your body to the place where the pose or movement feels a little uncomfortable. Not painful, not anything that will cause injury, but something that you're not entirely certain you're going to be able to manage. In grief, you feel that edge and continue to push at it with movement and stillness. This is how you find balance.

EVOLUTION TECHNIQUES AND EXERCISES

The following exercises and techniques are designed to help you evolve from heartbreak into living life fully. In the previous steps in the cycle, we have honored being present to the sadness, anger, regret, guilt, or shame. As we move forward, we can also acknowledge our courage, joy, balance, and perseverance. These exercises and techniques embody how to evolve from the darkness into the light.

Energy Burst

———

Grief is exhausting. This powerful exercise gives you a burst of oxygen in your body, lungs, and brain. It is meant to invigorate and inspire you to move through the darkness and to find the resilience and perseverance to embrace life after loss.

1. From a comfortable seated position, sit up straight so that your shoulders are over your hips. Interlace your fingers and extend your hands with straight arms in front of you.

2. As you inhale, lift your arms above your head. As you exhale, bring your arms down.

3. Repeat this motion in time with your breath, and pump oxygen into your heart. Choose whatever pace feels comfortable or desired, moving quickly and more strongly, or slowly and more gently. Let this match the pace at which you wish to move in your life. For more energy, do it faster and with more vigor.

4. Continue for two to three minutes. When you're ready, relax and come back to your natural breath.

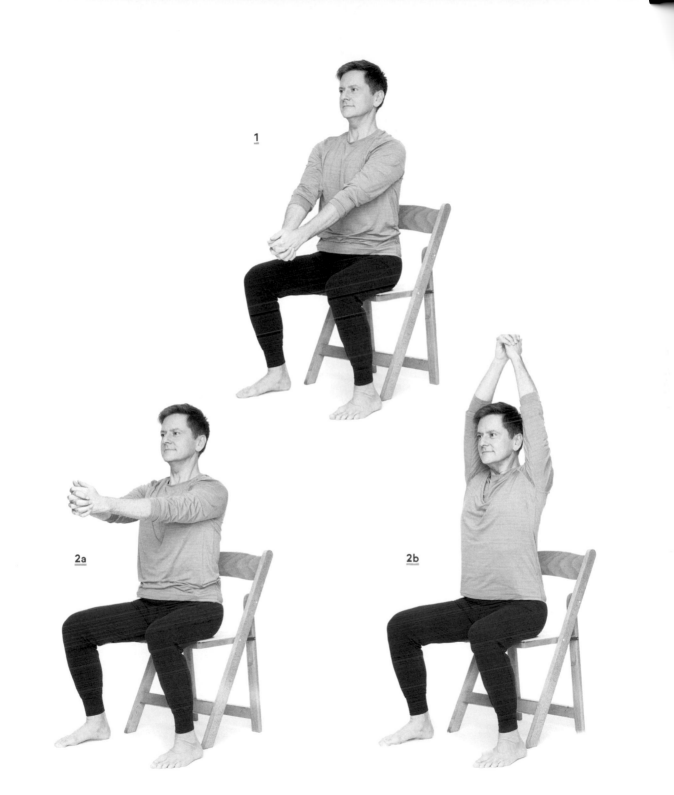

Maestro Breath

———

Within the devastation of loss, we often feel powerless, as though we have no control over our own lives. Maestro Breath helps you to orchestrate and master your energy flow and oxygen as you evolve toward liberation. It helps you to flow in your life again.

1. From a standing position, touch your thumb and index finger on each hand.

2. In a sequence, inhale quickly three times through your nose. On the first inhale, bring both hands, fingers touching, toward your chest; on the second, extend both hands away from your chest; and on the third inhale, bring both hands back to your chest.

3. As you exhale, release your hands and fingers behind you and shout, "HA!"

4. Repeat this gesture at your own pace for one to three minutes. Move your hands in and out, in time with your breath, as if you were leading an orchestra, and end each exhale with a shouted "HA!" When you're ready, relax and come back to your natural breath.

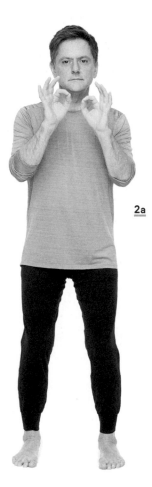

2a

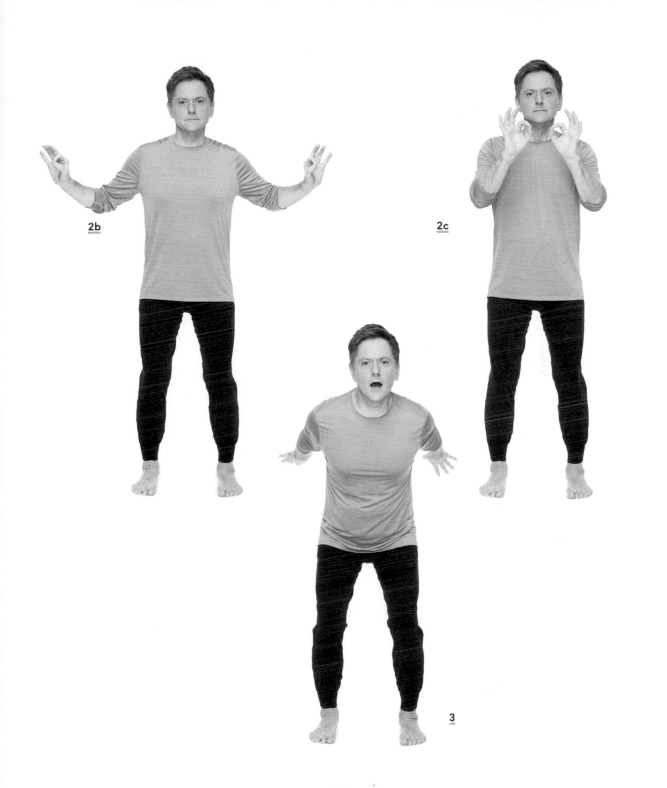

2b

2c

3

197

Breath of Courage

Moving forward in life, you will experience moments of doubt or fear. This exercise helps you embrace a powerful breath that connects to your courage and resilience. It connects you to your *roar* to empower and move you forward in your deepest struggle.

1. From a standing position, feet parallel and hip-width apart, bend your knees and lower your hips slightly.

2. Inhale deeply as you reach your arms up over your head.

3. As you exhale, bring your elbows toward your ribs with a powerful "HA!" Embody courage and strength.

4. Repeat this movement and breath at your own pace, five to ten times. Let your power guide you. When you're ready, release and relax your body; shake it out. Come back to your natural breath and stand in your power.

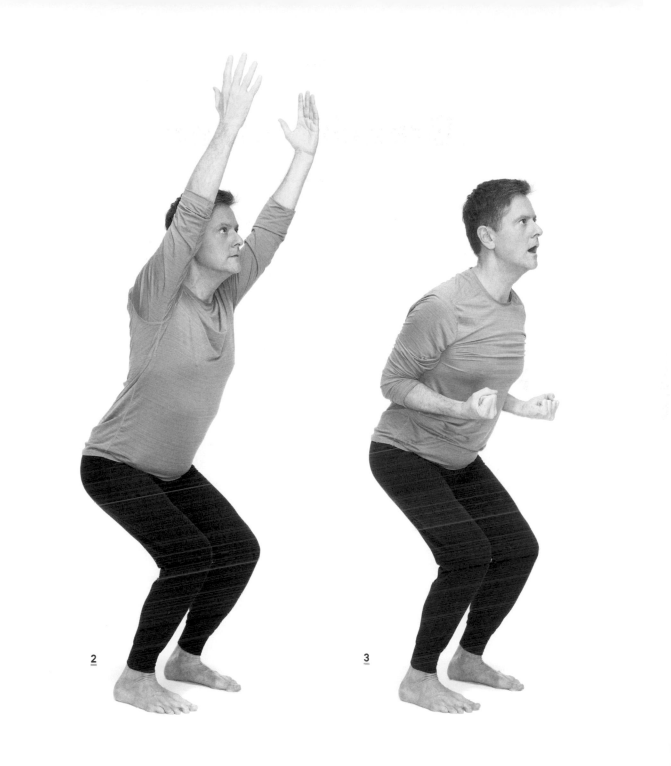

2

3

Breaking Open

———

Grief can leave us feeling stuck and trapped in suffering. This exercise accepts the reality of the struggle but provides an empowering way to push back and break through the pain. It helps release tightness to break open the heart and the throat so that we can reconnect to life and perseverance. Embrace your strength and worth. Choose to say yes to life, even within the devastation.

1. From a comfortable seated or standing position, bring both elbows close together in front of your chest at shoulder level, forearms raised, hands clenched into tight fists, as if they were in handcuffs.

2. Inhale deeply, and as you exhale, push both elbows out to the side, keeping your fists directly over your elbows, and shout, "HA!"

3. As you inhale, bring your elbows back to the original position, together in front of your chest, and as you exhale, push them away and shout, "HA!"

4. Repeat this sequence at your own pace for one to three minutes. When you're ready, relax your arms and come back to your natural breath.

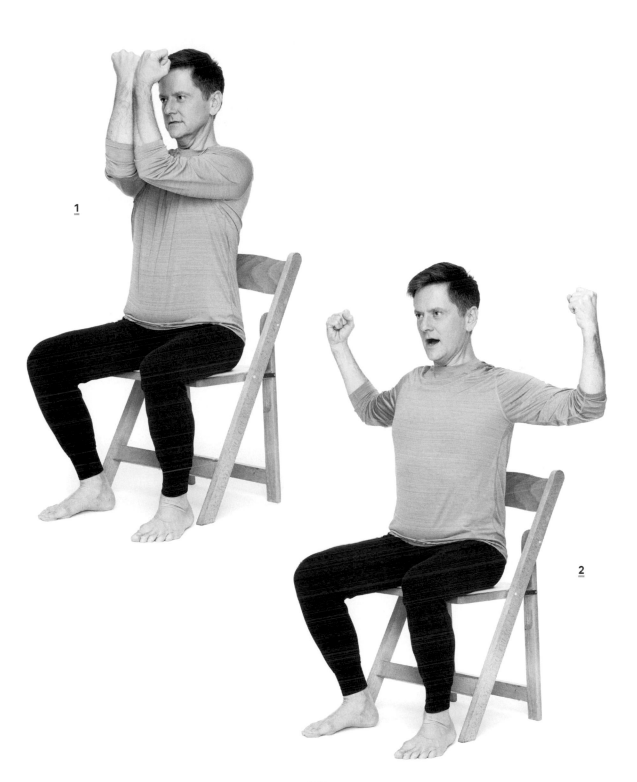

Warrior Spark

In moving through loss and pain, you are bowing to grief and a broken heart. This technique will ignite a flame to rejuvenate yourself as you move forward through your struggle. Recognize that you are still alive and you can choose to be a warrior of love.

1. From a standing position, widen your stance with your feet outside of your hips. With your heels in and your toes out, lower your hips with your knees above your heels and your hands at your sides.

2. Inhale, reach your arms up over your head, and tighten your fists above you. Exhale and bring your elbows down to the ribs with a powerful breath.

3. Repeat this sequence at your own pace. Use a powerful breath and the sound "HA!" to tap into your courage and strength.

4. Continue three to eight more times, then return to a natural standing position as you ignite your spark within.

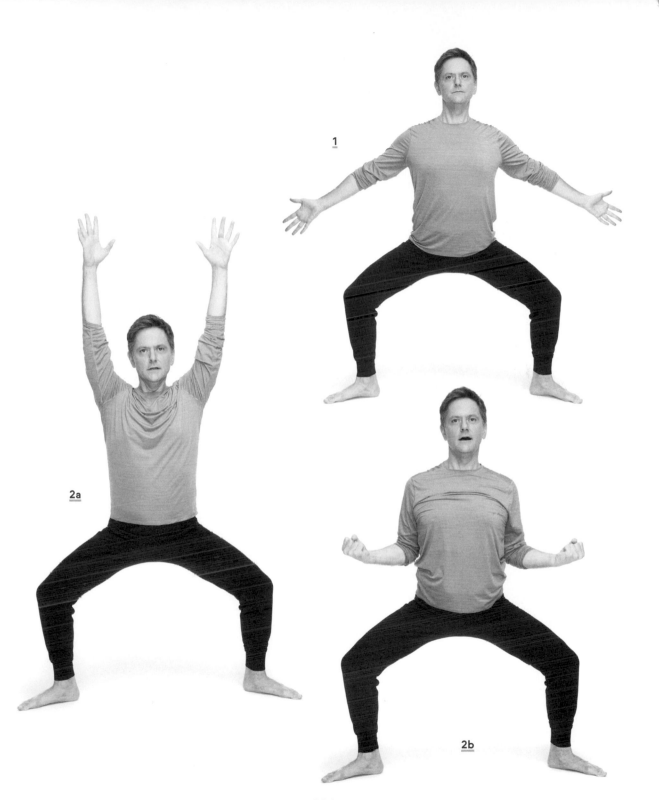

1

2a

2b

Hope in Action

The Hope in Action technique helps us flow forward from heartbreak. It allows us to visualize better days to come. This exercise helps you evolve and develop perseverance as you move toward hope.

1. From a comfortable seated or standing position, place your elbows by your ribs and hold your hands in gentle fists.

2. While staying in one place, and without moving your legs, pump your arms forward and back, fists in front of you, as if you were running in place.

3. Gaze at one still object in front of you. As you focus on that object, imagine that it is something specific you're running toward in your life, something you are trying to manifest. See the future you want as complete. See yourself writing it. Creating it. Collaborating with others to make it happen. Connect to the emotional space, time, and vision to manifest it. Find the passion in it.

4. Continue at your own pace, moving your hands forward and back as if running, for three to five minutes. When finished, relax your arms and rest.

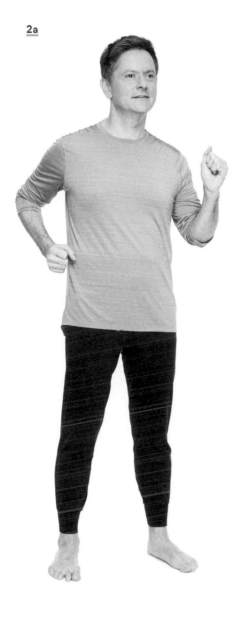

2a

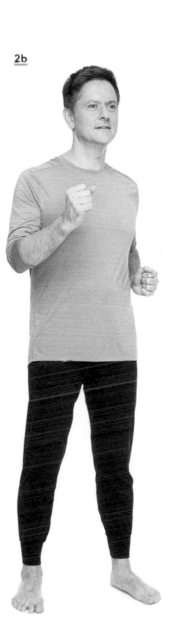

2b

Laughing Gas

In the depths of sadness or depression, we can perhaps believe that happiness is no longer possible. Laughing Gas embraces laughter as a tool for healing. Laughter can be medicine. Allowing yourself to laugh doesn't deny your loss or sadness; it helps move trapped emotions through and out of your body. Whatever you're feeling, laughter can release it.

1. From a comfortable seated or standing position, bring your cupped hands in front of your mouth and inhale through your nose. Breathe in as much oxygen as possible. Imagine that it's laughing gas.

2. As you exhale, release your hands, and allow laughter to come through your mouth. If the laughter doesn't feel natural or organic, do it anyway until, ideally, genuine laughter comes on its own.

3. Repeat the sequence, inhaling through cupped hands, removing your hands, and exhaling laughter. Connect to whatever you're feeling in the moment, and allow laughter to help guide it through. For instance, if you feel uncomfortable, express an uncomfortable laugh; if angry or sad, express an angry or sad laugh. Observe whether your laughter shifts.

4. Continue at your own pace for a few minutes, or at least two to four times.

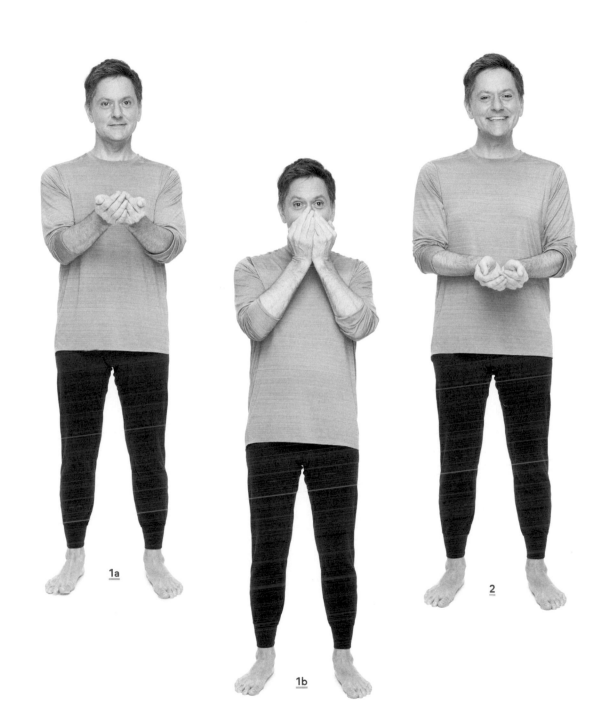

1a

1b

2

207

Mistake Laughter

———

We're all human and make mistakes, but we're so cruel to ourselves when we do. This playful technique allows us some grace to be able to laugh about our mistakes.

1. From a comfortable seated or standing position, inhale and bring your hand up to your mouth. Gasp like you made a big mistake, then exhale and release your hand to your side with a laugh. You are choosing to laugh about your mistake instead of beating yourself up.

2. Repeat two to four more times, then come back to your natural breath and observe how you feel.

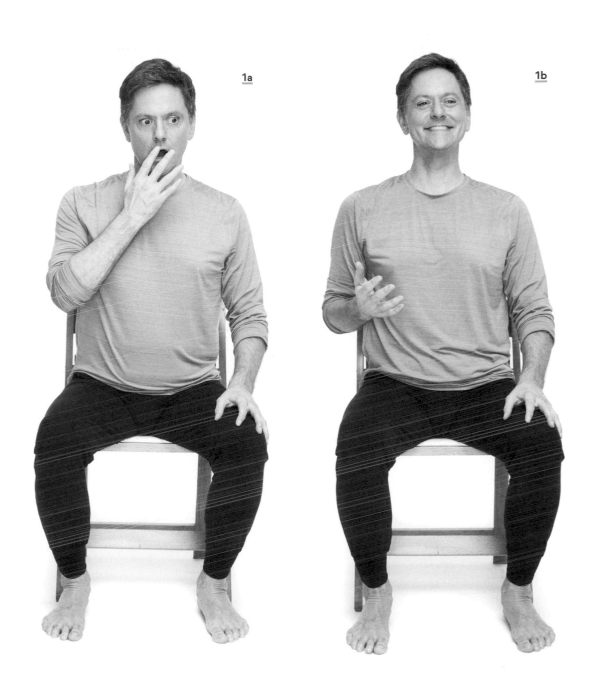

Body Judgment Laughter

Body insecurity and shame is something that many people experience. This technique is designed to address and accept all areas of your body that you judge. It uses laughter to shift negative perceptions to help you embrace your body.

1. From a comfortable seated or standing position, place your hand on an area of your body that you're insecure about, and then laugh about it. You can allow the laughter to be fake at first.

2. Place your hand on another area of your body that you criticize and judge, and then laugh about it.

3. Continue in this way with different parts of your body, and whatever emotion comes up, use laughter to move it through. Even if the laughter is fake, observe how the laughter shifts your perception after you've done it a few times. This may take a while to get into, but it can be liberating in overcoming body shame.

4. Continue at your own pace for one to two minutes. This is a path to accepting and loving your body just as it is.

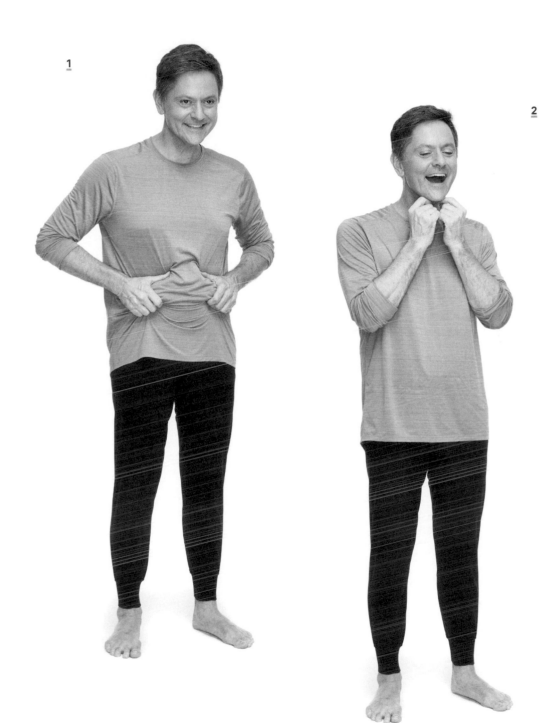

Open Heart Laughter

You can honor your grief and also honor happiness. Remember, happiness is your birthright, and you deserve to be happy despite your tragedies and losses. Laughter can help to shift the pain a little. This is hope. Your heart is strong, and it can heal.

1. From a comfortable seated or standing position, inhale deeply and bring both hands over your heart.

2. As you exhale, open your hands wide to the side like wings and laugh. If the laughter doesn't feel authentic, do it anyway until, ideally, genuine laughter emerges.

3. Repeat at your own pace for a few minutes. Allow your laughter to open and heal your heart.

SMALL SHIFT

With these laughing exercises, I'm not suggesting that you will suddenly be happy *right now*, one-two-three go! Happiness doesn't work like that. These are *practices*. You may not be happy before you do them, but by doing them, you might feel just a little bit happier. That small shift can serve as evidence that you still have the ability to feel happiness.

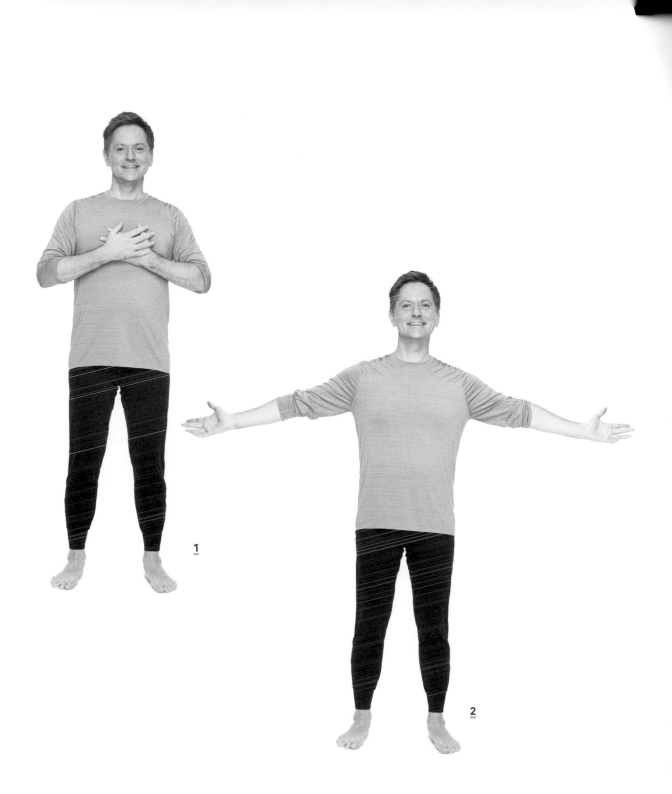

1

2

213

Pendulum

———

This practice intentionally tests your balance, so that you must continually find stability and balance, both in the moment and within the flow of life. Grief can knock us to the ground, and with Pendulum, we can recognize this and acknowledge it. You may at first feel stable, until suddenly you are not. If you fall, that's normal. Just be aware that despite the tragedy you've been through, you always continue to move.

1. From a standing position, hands at your sides, shift your weight to your left foot, and slightly flex your right foot, so it isn't bearing any weight.

2. As you inhale, swing your right leg forward, keeping it straight, raising it as far as you can. Then as you exhale, swing your right leg back, extending it behind you as far as you can.

3. Continue at your own pace for two to three minutes. Inhale and swing your right leg forward; exhale and swing it back, like a pendulum. Each time, try to swing farther while maintaining your balance; if you fall, simply start over. Allow your hands to move as they will, and imagine your left foot rooted into the earth.

4. Repeat on the other side, shifting your weight to your right foot and swinging your left leg like a pendulum, moving forward and backward with your breath.

5. Continue at your own pace for two to three minutes, then relax.

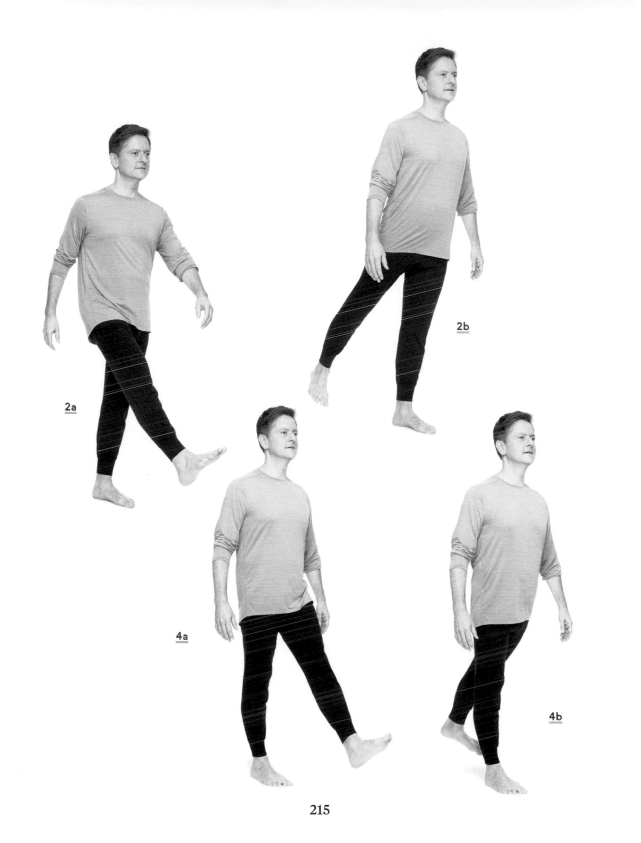

2a

2b

4a

4b

215

Tree

___

In grief, we can get stuck in our head and become disconnected from our body. Tree posture allows you to get out of your head and ground yourself into your deep roots, to find a steadiness of support. Some days your balance will be better than others. It is easy to adjust this posture to find and maintain balance, depending on your level of ability. Choose what supports you.

1. From a standing position, bend your right knee and place the sole of your right foot on your left leg, either at the thigh, calf, or ankle. Lower positions are easier to balance. In addition, focusing on one still object in front of you can help you maintain balance. If keeping your foot raised is too difficult, place the right heel on the left ankle, and touch the floor with your right toes, as if it were a kickstand. Bring your palms together in prayer position in front of your heart.

2. Connect to your breath, and feel your left leg rooted in the earth. If you wish, raise your hands to the sky as if they were branches. Hold for a minute, or as long as you want.

3. Repeat on the other side, standing on your right leg, lifting and placing your left foot, and holding while observing your breath.

4. Continue for a minute or longer. If you fall before you're ready, simply restore your position. When finished, stand with your hands at your sides, and observe your breath.

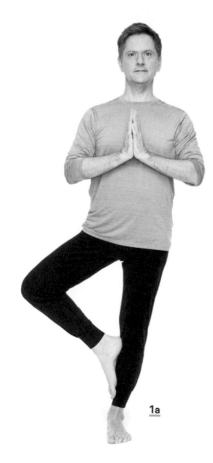

1a

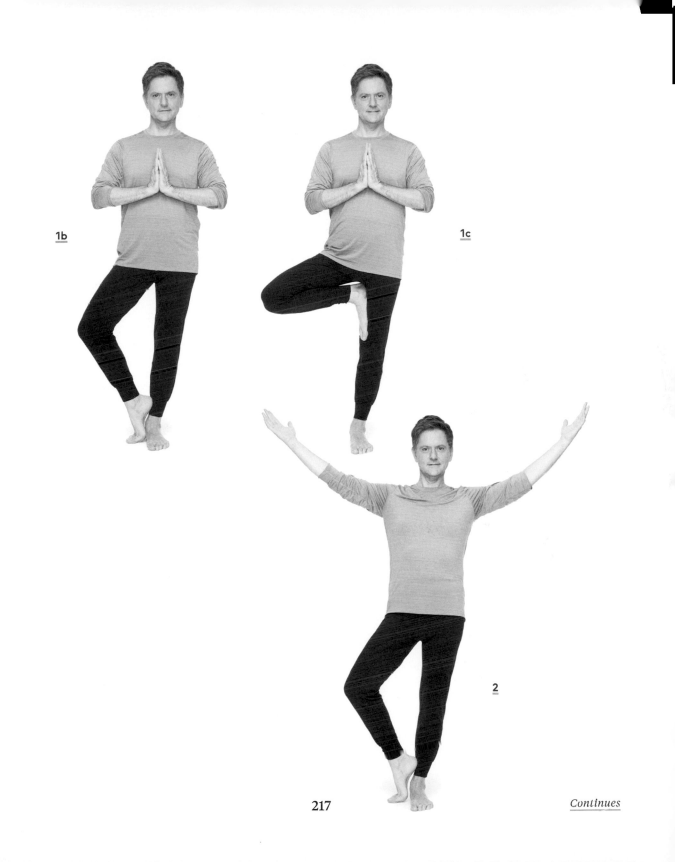

1b

1c

2

Continues

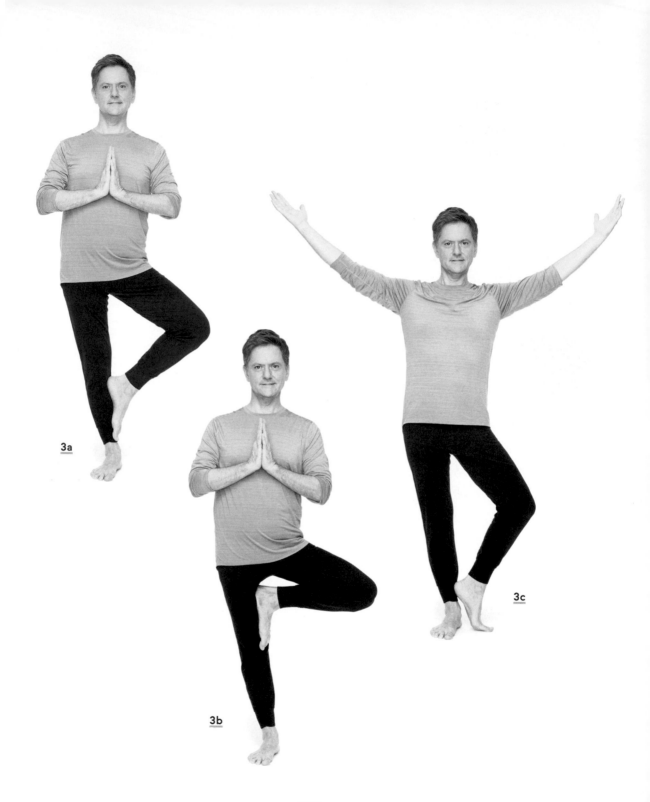

3a

3b

3c

218

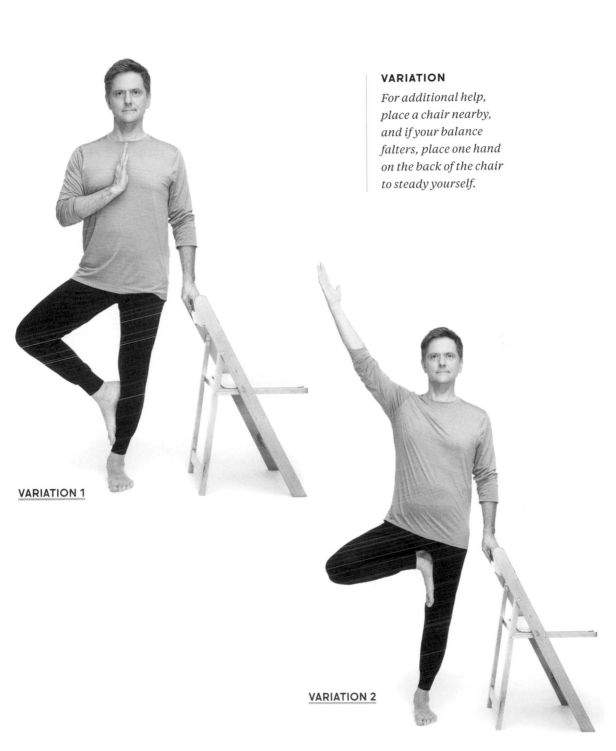

VARIATION

For additional help, place a chair nearby, and if your balance falters, place one hand on the back of the chair to steady yourself.

VARIATION 1

VARIATION 2

219

Alternate-Nostril Breathing

———

This breathing technique balances the breathing between the right and left nostril, right and left brain, right and left lungs, and right and left sides of the body. It helps bring more awareness to your breath, while clearing and quieting the mind and reducing anxiety. Breathing in and out of the right nostril provides energy; breathing in and out of the left nostril instills calm. We need both, always.

1. From a comfortable seated position, place your left hand on your left knee and lift your right hand to your nose.

2. Exhale fully, and close your right nostril with your right thumb. Inhale fully through your left nostril, and then close your left nostril with your fingers while opening your right nostril by releasing your thumb.

3. Exhale fully through your right nostril, and then also inhale fully through the right nostril.

4. Close the right nostril with the thumb while opening the left nostril by releasing your fingers, and then exhale and inhale fully through the left nostril.

5. Close the left nostril with your fingers, release your thumb from the right nostril, and exhale and inhale fully from your right nostril.

6. Continue this sequence of alternate-nostril breathing for up to five minutes. Finish the practice by exhaling completely on the left side, then come back to your natural breath.

2a

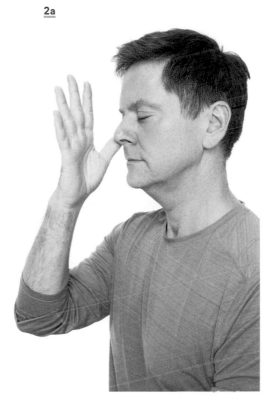

2b

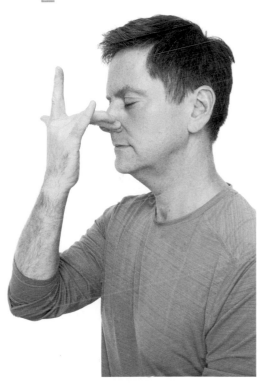

Evolving Self

This exercise is a guided meditation that is meant to inspire reflection. As you recall your own perseverance in the face of life's obstacles, this sparks your ability to overcome the loss you face now and transition from darkness to the hope of new beginnings.

1. **Embody the wound:** Assume Child's Pose (page 54) or Fetal Position (page 173). Imagine you are a womb that is about to give birth. Recall a time in your past when you felt broken, either physically, spiritually, or emotionally. Locate where the place of feeling broken lives in your mind and body. Focus on it. Exaggerate the physical, spiritual, and emotional aspects of the wound. Connect to your feelings of being broken. Breathe and embody the struggle.

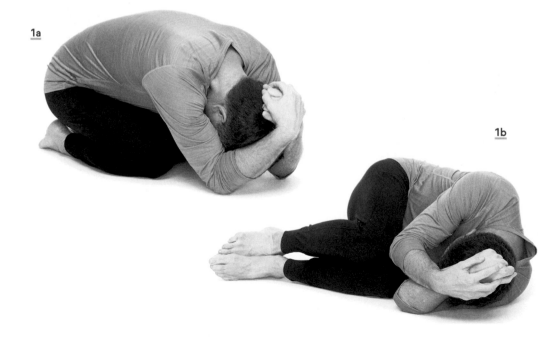

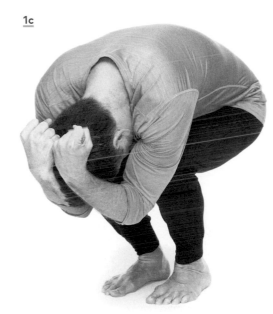

1c

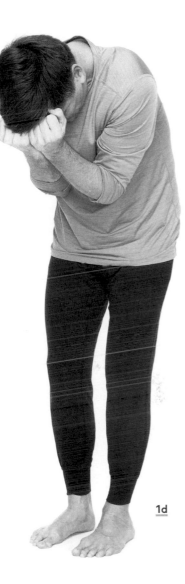

1d

223

Continues

2. **What happened next:** Inquire within and consider what happened next. How did you move forward? What did you learn about yourself from that time? What personal resource was discovered? What helped you in your struggle and suffering?

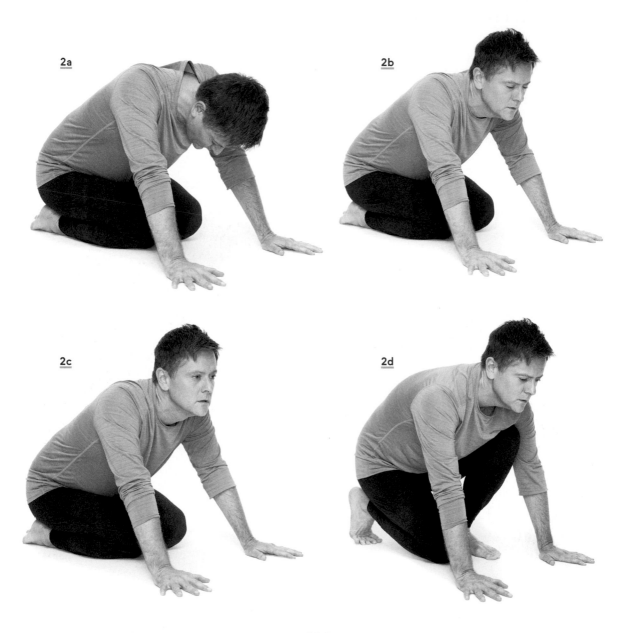

2a

2b

2c

2d

3. **Take a stand:** In order to embody moving away from the pain of the past, stand up from your position on the floor. Then perform a modified version of Love Taps (page 117). Lightly tap your body all over with open palms, tapping your legs, back, butt, stomach, chest, heart, arms, neck, and head. As you lightly tap all over your body, say, "I am . . . ," and complete the sentence with something positive to help awaken your perseverance and resilience. It could be, "I am courageous," "I am strong," or "I am powerful." Tap yourself back into life with powerful affirmations to help you push through your fear.

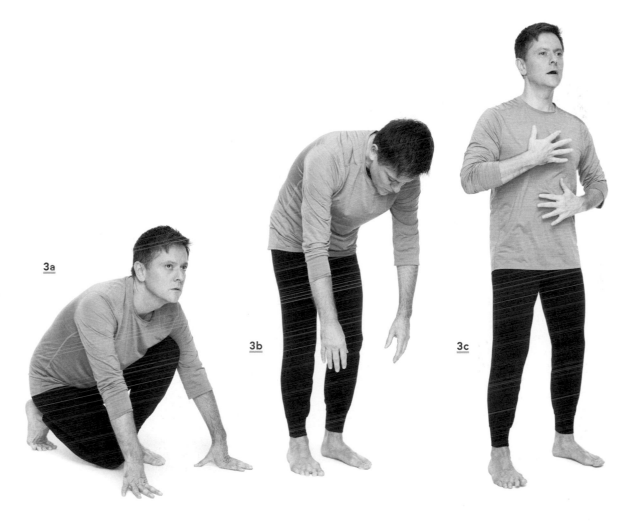

3a

3b

3c

Continues

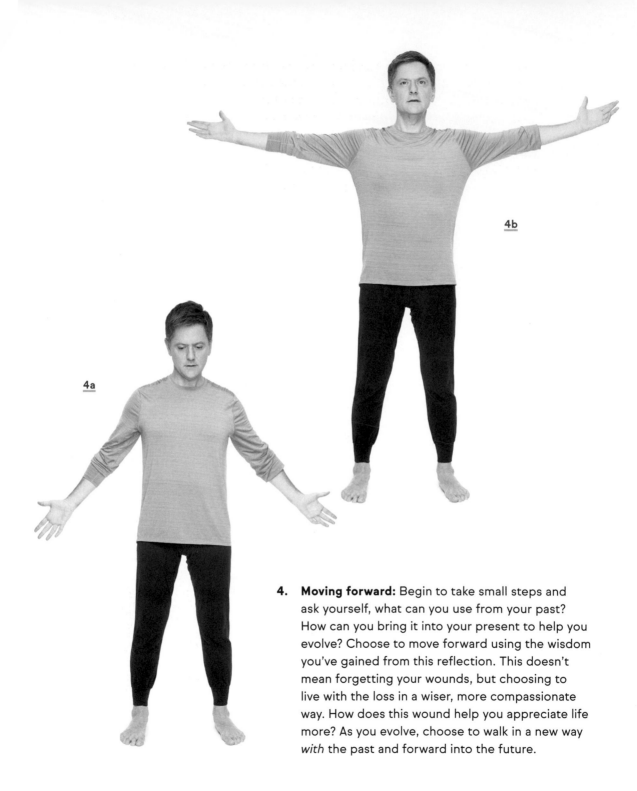

4a

4b

4. **Moving forward:** Begin to take small steps and ask yourself, what can you use from your past? How can you bring it into your present to help you evolve? Choose to move forward using the wisdom you've gained from this reflection. This doesn't mean forgetting your wounds, but choosing to live with the loss in a wiser, more compassionate way. How does this wound help you appreciate life more? As you evolve, choose to walk in a new way *with* the past and forward into the future.

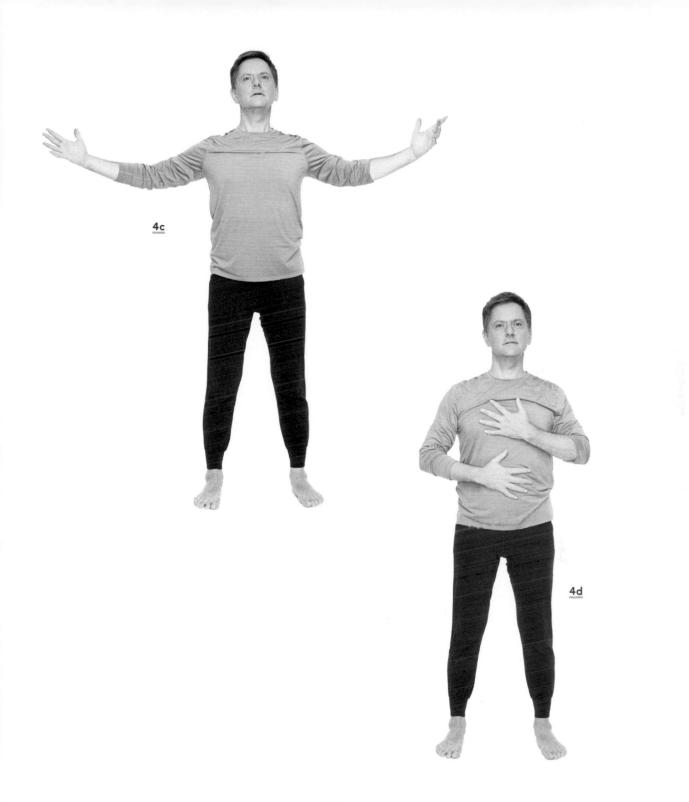

4c

4d

Star Warrior

This warrior flow helps you connect to your empowerment as you evolve through fear and struggle. It helps you find the strength to move forward through your pain with grace. It allows you to connect to your body as you flow and evolve toward perseverance and courage. You are alive for a reason. Star Warrior helps you to expand, to take up space in life, and to recognize that you matter.

1. From a standing position, move into the yoga pose known as Warrior Two: Widen your feet, and point your right toes to the right, while bending your right knee and keeping it over your right heel. Straighten your left leg behind you, with your back foot parallel to the back edge of your mat, and point your left foot slightly forward. Extend your arms level at shoulder height and over your legs, forward and backward, as you look over your right arm and leg. Keep your shoulders centered over your hips.

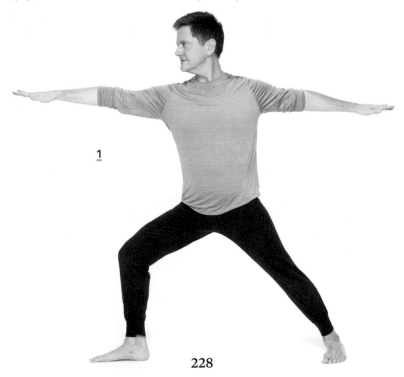

1

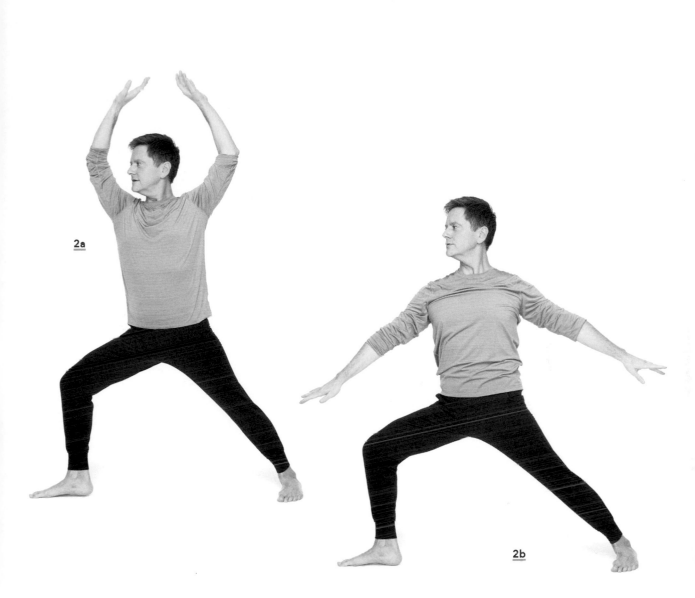

2a

2b

2. As you inhale, reach your arms up like wings, and as you exhale, bring them down. Repeat this gesture at your own pace for one to two minutes—inhaling your wings up, exhaling your wings down. As you flow with grace, connect to the earth beneath you. Connect to the resilient warrior that lives within.

Continues

3. When you're ready, shift to the Star pose. Straighten both legs and face front, with your heels pointed inward and your toes pointed out. Lift your arms, keeping them straight, with palms up, into a V. Your whole body will be shaped like an X. Hold this pose for one to two minutes, breathing deeply, as you connect to these affirmations: *I matter. My life matters. I take up space. I'm alive.*

4. On an exhale, return to the Warrior Two pose but on the other side: Face your left leg, bend your left knee over your left heel, keep your right leg straight and back with toes slightly turned in, and stretch your arms outward at shoulder height, left arm forward and right arm back.

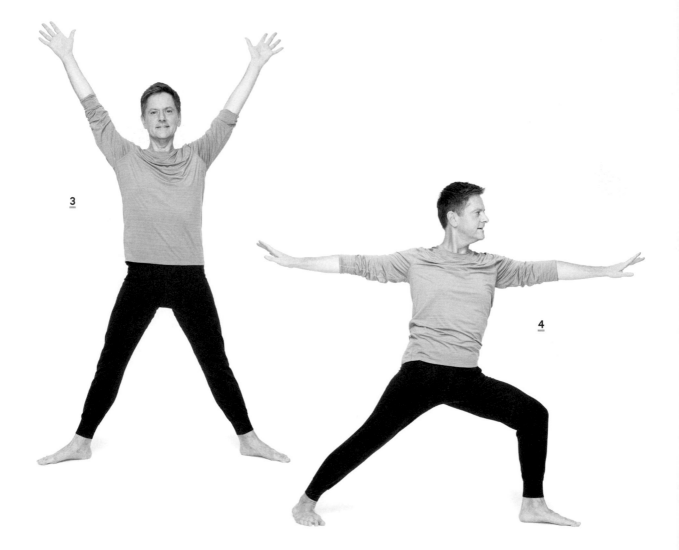

3

4

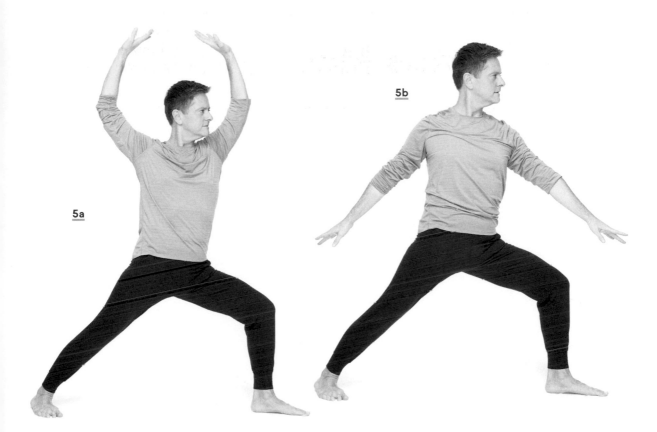

5a

5b

5. Repeat the wing-like motion in step 2. As you inhale, lift your arms up, and as you exhale, float them down.

6. Repeat the entire sequence again. Continue at your own pace for two to four minutes, then relax. Connect to the graceful warrior within.

Lotus Meditation

———

The Lotus Meditation helps to move us from darkness to light. You can open your flower buds. You can rise up and honor your loss. Love still remains within you. Honor it by sharing it with the world. This meditation does not have numbered steps; once you begin, the meditation follows your thoughts, lasts as long as you want, and ends whenever you feel ready or complete.

1. From a comfortable seated position, bring the base of your palms together at your heart center. Touch your thumbs and pinky fingers together. Open the rest of your fingers like a lotus flower opening toward the sunlight.

2. Close your eyes and take several long deep breaths. Then meditate on what represents the roots that ground and support you. Do you receive nourishment from faith, family, loved ones, or friends so you can keep opening up to the sun? If you find it difficult to feel the sun, what nourishes your roots in murky times?

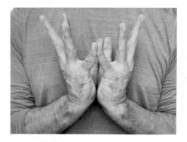

3. Here are some further thoughts to consider in your meditation:

    *   Know that your joy can live through grief.
    *   Identify and experience your loss, and consider how you have grown through it.
    *   Are you more open to love? Do you appreciate love more?
    *   Try shifting from the negative pain of the past and open yourself to any positive hopes and desires you have in the present or feel for the future.
    *   Feel the longing for your heart to open.
    *   Dwell in your positive experiences. Listen to the longing of your heart and your desire to keep growing. Ground yourself in your longing.
    *   Recognize that you are alive and growing.

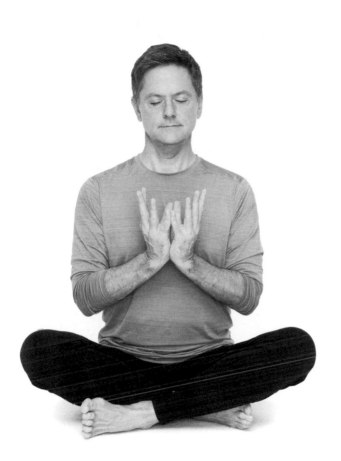

RISE ABOVE

Without mud, there would be no lotus flower. Making use of the sludge, the lotus grows and blooms into a beautiful and fragrant flower. The blossoms close their petals at night and reopen in the morning sun. There is constant resurgence and renewal, a reinvention of expression. Even in a muddy and difficult environment, lotus blossoms move forward and express their unique beauty. This muddy existence is a gift for the lotus, as their roots draw in sustenance from the murky waters below to sustain the flower.

In your dark night of the soul, allow yourself some grace. Push away the pain of the world and find safety in a protective inner cocoon. Even when you close your buds to find renewal, life continues, and once you've rested, you can find the courage to slowly reopen to life. Hope for brighter days. Believe that your suffering will bring deeper meaning into your life. Even though the muck feels like quicksand, you can rise above the suffering.

Moving into Transformation

This book has provided many exercises and techniques to help you move through your loss and pain. Let's identify your struggle and guide you in a transformative ritual to achieve a specific result.

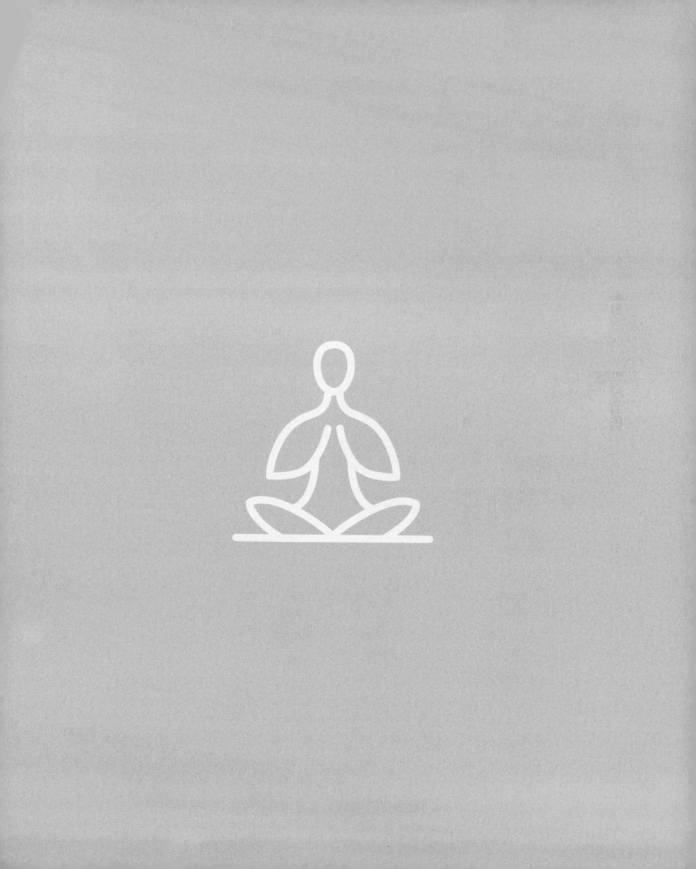

6

Transformation

Yoga does not just change the way we see things,
it transforms the person who sees.

—B.K.S. IYENGAR

Transformation is the process of life. When you're feeling devastated by loss and heartbreak, it's possible to move forward with intention and purpose. This book has provided many tools and techniques to help you move through pain. Let's blend these techniques and exercises together to create a ritual to move from darkness to light. Let's honor loss and struggle so we can grow from the ruins into something else.

One thing is for certain: Change is inevitable. In life, things are continually transforming. Change is all around us and always has been. Every season transforms into another season. We continually transform: We begin as an embryo and we are born. A baby transforms into a toddler. A toddler transforms into a child, a child becomes a teenager, and a teenager becomes an adult. We grow and eventually die. Even death is a transformation of our physical body.

We want to think of transformation as a good thing so we can become better or greater. We want to transform from the cocoon into the butterfly. But bad things are also transformative. Tragedy can cause posttraumatic stress that shuts us down. A breakup or betrayal can leave us feeling hurt. An accident or disease can transform our personal health in compromising ways.

In early 2020, the Covid-19 pandemic disrupted lives all around the world. The rituals we used in the past to process loss, like gathering together in a ceremony, became dangerous. Instead of holding hands, lighting candles, and crying on someone's shoulder, we had to say goodbye to loved ones on FaceTime and attend Zoom funerals.

The grieving process was so disrupted, it became even more challenging to process loss. Funerals and burials aren't just for the deceased; they're also for the living. When we don't have our grief witnessed, it can create an immense emotional challenge, resulting in anxiety and depression. These negative effects can impact our physical and mental health and our immune systems, causing an increase in alcohol and substance abuse. This can make it hard to concentrate, and it disrupts our sleep patterns. These losses will no doubt cause delayed grief in many people. It is good to note that our grief knows when it is time to come down from the shelf for healing. Of course, when delayed grief hits, it never feels like it's a good time. But when it does come down, our job is to be present for it and not make it wrong for showing up.

While we may crave connecting with others, sometimes we are forced to isolate and grieve alone. This has been painful for so many as well as for me.

We all need help and support in our transformations. Even my practice is part of my own transformation. My own transformation would look quite different without the support of others.

In 2005, I had just completed my Heart Touch therapy training, which is a compassionate, sacred, gentle ritual of massage to the dying. The school connected me with Ida, a volunteer coordinator for hospice.

After we talked on the phone several times, we met. Even though she shared how much loss and death she had witnessed in her life, she still had a sweetness in her voice, an appreciation of life, and a passion for helping others.

Ida set me up with several people who were in hospice in their final weeks. The first time I sat with someone on their death bed, I felt the profoundness of the moment. I was scared and intimidated offering compassionate, loving Heart Touch in moments when their body was decaying. In that vulnerability, Ida was present with me, offering such kindness and support. She listened to my fears and reassured me that what I was feeling was normal.

Ida was a protective mama who made sure I was doing my work and practicing self-care. For her that included going to parties hosted by her volunteers; she was a lover of life and laughter. It was inspiring to get to know this woman whose job was to make sure no one died alone and without touch if they wanted it.

When Ida heard I was doing a new practice called Grief Yoga, she loved the concept and was so supportive. She connected me with the bereavement coordinator at a local hospice. That's when I started teaching to bereavement groups for those whose loved one had died. She connected me with other volunteer associations all over Southern California. Even after my Grief Yoga practice was flourishing, whenever she reached out to me and asked me to do Heart Touch with someone, I was there for her to do that.

Just as I was finishing this book, I found out that Ida had died on Christmas Day of Covid-19. Her loss was devastating. I had no idea Ida had Covid-19. I was told it was quick; two weeks after being diagnosed, she was gone. My heart sank. I wish I could have given Heart Touch to her while she was in the hospital. The woman who made sure others felt loved and cared for at the end of life was, like so many who died of Covid-19, alone and without friends or family at the end.

Loss is draining. Our minds can be scattered and chaotic. We need something to center our mind, body, and spirit.

I was Ida's yoga teacher, but she was also my teacher. Ida taught me how to be present, kind, and curious to those who are at the end of life. To meet them where they are. Her sweetness and service to others is part of my healing ritual, which I will take onward.

HEALING RITUALS

Rituals are powerful experiences that transform loss and struggle. Whether they are done individually or in a group, they can be a guide to help us move forward, to help us grow and heal.

Rituals are sacred ceremonies that consist of specific intentions and actions that are done according to a prescribed order. They are ceremonies that share what's important in our lives and express who we are. Gatherings like going to concerts and plays are ways to celebrate life. So are graduations and birthdays. We give a baby shower for pregnant women or say a prayer before Thanksgiving dinner. We hold hands, we bow our heads to say grace, and then we say amen.

Ram Dass said, "We are all just walking one another home." Public rituals include meaningful acts in our family, culture, religion, and spirituality. They help us connect with other people. We have funerals when people die to help mourners center themselves and find a way forward. When we gather one last time to honor someone who has died, we wear black, bring flowers, and share memories. In Christianity, we mourn and celebrate the deceased loved one being reunited with Jesus. In Judaism, people sit shiva, a seven-day mourning period, while Catholics hold a mass, and Muslims wash the body and shroud it in three sheets.

Private rituals can include almost anything: meditating during a specific time of day, writing in a journal, making your bed in the morning, going to the gym for a workout, or sitting down and reading a book. This is something we do to bring order, keep centered, and stay fit when we're feeling overwhelmed.

Loss is draining. Our minds can be scattered and chaotic. We need something to center our mind, body, and spirit. We light a candle next to a picture of a loved one who has died to honor that love and to express how much we miss them. These rituals can be challenging. You may wonder why you need to set aside focused time to feel the pain. Grief and loss deserve time. The pain is asking for attention. Delving into loss, grief, and trauma is an active way to acknowledge all you have been through. You're taking some space to feel and breathe and remember the love.

I created Grief Yoga as a ritual to honor loss. It is a sacred space to transform pain and struggle. We look into another person's eyes and witness their grief, and we also look within because it's important to accept reality. When we can't process our losses with other people, the intensity of our grief can get suppressed and delayed. Grief needs dedicated time and space or it can go on for decades. I encourage you to create your own rituals to express and acknowledge your grief.

A ritual has a beginning, middle, and end. Stacy, a client of mine who was grieving the betrayal of her boyfriend, wrote him a letter describing her hurt and pain. She never sent the letter, but instead, she gathered pictures of the two of them and burned them and the letter. It helped her to create a ritual to express her pain to let go.

When you are creating a personal private ritual, do what's comfortable for you and make it your own. Here are some things to consider:

- Designate a specific time and place.
- Think of actions that symbolize your feelings.
- Ring a bell at the beginning and at the end. This will help you enter and exit the sacred space consciously.
- Light a candle.
- Say a prayer.
- Read an inspiring poem.
- Sing a song or play music.
- Write a letter about your pain and struggle.

You might sit quietly through the whole ritual and not move at all, and that's perfect, too.

If you get frustrated or confused along the way, just be curious and keep focused on why you're doing this.

TRANSFORMATIVE FLOWS

Grief Yoga includes transformative flows that are inspired by kriyas. *Kriya* is a term that means "completed action." It is a specific set of exercises—including breathing techniques, sound, mantras, and physical poses—that are used to unlock energy channels or chakras in the body. Like rituals, we practice the sequence to achieve a specific outcome. Kriyas are meant to enable subtle and direct changes in the mind and body to help lift the spirit. The intention is to heal and enlighten someone in their struggle.

Consider practicing the sequences below as if they were classes; these will help when you feel anxious, sad, angry, regretful, afraid, or depressed. They will guide you through your stuck emotions and create a path toward a lighter state of being. They will help center you, mentally and physically, as you create newer and healthier patterns. They will ground you and gently move your spine to help create a fire within you. They will open your heart and allow love to blossom. They will open your throat and liberate your voice. Most importantly, they will help you find union among mind, body, and spirit.

Each transformational ritual begins with a journaling prompt to help center you. This is a time to explore and express your pain and struggle through words. Write out whatever criticism or hurt you're experiencing.

After the journaling prompt, explore and identify the reason you're doing this sequence. Explore your intention and your motivation, or what you hope to achieve. When you connect to why, or the reason beneath the goal, it can help set you up for success. For example, if you're focused on "releasing pent-up anger," perhaps your intention could be "to channel my anger into something passionate and positive for myself and others." If you are feeling depressed, your intention could be "to find more enjoyment and experience the many different emotions of life."

Then allow the movement experience to shift the pain. Take your time within the process, and remember, if there's any physical pain, pull back and rest. If there's an emotional struggle, move forward and focus on what you can release.

The reflections for "moving forward" are tools to help you achieve your desired result. They are affirmations, journaling prompts, healthy habits, or ways to find deeper connections. Apply what resonates best for you.

If you get frustrated or confused along the way, just be curious and stay focused on why you're doing this. What motivates you within this transformation? Allow your intention to guide your path to release and move through the struggle. Approach this process from a beginner's mind and with deep compassion.

Transform Anger Into Purpose

―――

The yoga mat is an ideal space to embrace anger with mindfulness and compassion. Emotions create movement and anger has many aspects. When you experience injustice, anger can help you recognize that changes need to happen. You can use anger as motivation to find clarity, to alter circumstances, and to create boundaries when someone is threatening you. Anger can be useful when you're feeling disrespected, abused, or when you just can't take it anymore. When you're in danger, it creates an adrenaline rush, a spark of energy that activates strength. When anger is simmering, it can burn us up. When you step into your anger, however, it can help you find the will to live through grief. It can inspire you to take action when you need to push through something and get it done.

JOURNALING PROMPTS

I'm angry at . . .

When I'm angry, I . . .

Anger feels like . . .

When I'm angry, my body feels like . . .

INTENTION

My intention is . . .

MOVING FORWARD

Write a letter: Address the letter to who or what you're angry at. Don't hold back; release all your angry thoughts and feelings. When it's complete, witness your pain. Find compassion for yourself. Then throw the letter away.

Take a walk: Reflect on these questions:

What is my anger here to teach me?

What does it want me to change?

What can I do to transform my anger into something positive?

Repeat this affirmation: I can feel my anger and still stay in control. I choose to stop taking things personally and let go.

TRANSFORMATIVE FLOW

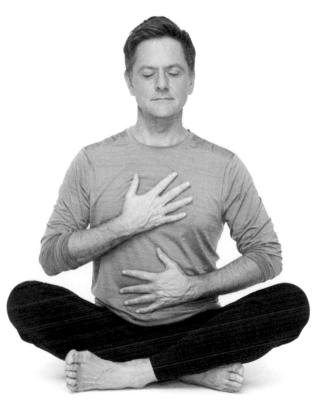

Transform Sadness into Love

———

We all experience heartbreak. Loss is universal, and grief exists because our world is constantly changing. The law of nature teaches us that things come and go. The nature of life is impermanence. Loss is inevitable and constant. Whatever is going on right now, good or bad, this too shall pass.

Sometimes change can be exciting. We like it when good things come that enhance our lives. But when we become attached to things and they leave, we experience grief. Remember that crying is a natural part of healing when you're heartbroken and lonely, longing for what you're missing, and yearning for the way things were. Grief is here to help heal the pain; it's a quiet energy that can nurture a broken heart.

To process grief, you have to feel it. Feel your disappointment, fear, and sadness. Connect to where you're feeling these emotions in your body. Instead of thinking about it, surrender to the feeling.

JOURNALING PROMPTS

The reason I'm sad is . . .

My heart feels . . .

When I'm sad, my body feels like . . .

INTENTION

My intention is . . .

MOVING FORWARD

Take a walk: When you are walking, reflect on your loved one. Feel them beside you, supporting you. Whisper to them, "I'm sending you love. I'm sending you my love. I'm sending you love. I'm sending you my love."

Write a letter to your loved one: In a letter, describe a memory you will always cherish, and share how deeply the person affected your life.

Create something: Express your love by creating something, whether that's a drawing, a meal that reminds you of them, or a scrapbook of memories.

Repeat this affirmation: In my sadness, I love myself and my beloved.

TRANSFORMATIVE FLOW

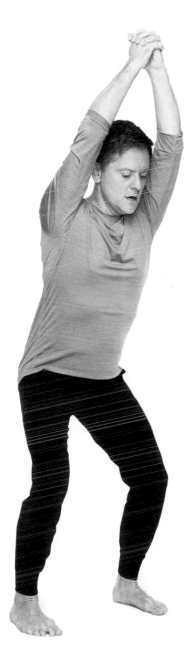

Transform Fear into Courage

Fear can come from feeling overwhelmed, anxious, and confused. It can stem from trauma. At the same time, it can bring more stability and security to our life and protect us from danger. If we embrace a healthy fear, it can connect us to the peace and security we desire. If fear cripples us, it can make us feel stuck.

We have the ability to move beyond our fear with courage. We can change and grow to help express what we want and need. The following sequence of exercises is focused on facing our fears so we can handle things better. This empowering class will boost your self-confidence and self-esteem so you can shift your fear into love.

JOURNALING PROMPT

I'm afraid of . . .

What scares me the most is . . .

When I'm afraid, my body feels like . . .

INTENTION

My intention is . . .

MOVING FORWARD

List your fears: When you're done writing, tear the list up, declaring, "You have no power over me."

Take a walk and reflect: As you walk, ask yourself: What's one thing I can do today to face my fear?

Repeat this affirmation: I am willing to release my fearful ideas from my mind, body, and spirit. I accept what I cannot change, and I have the courage to change the things I can.

TRANSFORMATIVE FLOW

Transform Guilt into Grace

———

We feel guilt when we act outside of our accepted belief system. When we feel we've done something wrong, guilt reminds us to learn from our mistakes and take responsibility as we move forward. It's a moral compass to help us live with more integrity. It teaches us to learn from our mistakes and to avoid making further ones in the future. If guilt isn't addressed and expressed, we feel like hiding. We feel shame.

JOURNALING PROMPT

Write about a time when you did something you thought was wrong.

I feel guilty about . . .

What if I had . . .

If only I hadn't . . .

I should have . . .

When I'm in guilt or regret, my body feels like . . .

INTENTION

My intention is . . .

MOVING FORWARD

Write yourself a note: List the areas in which you judge or criticize yourself. What is your guilt here to teach you?

Connect with someone you trust: Share your guilt with a confidant. Do you need to make amends with anyone?

Repeat this affirmation: I am willing to forgive myself and others. I let go of the mistakes of the past.

TRANSFORMATIVE FLOW

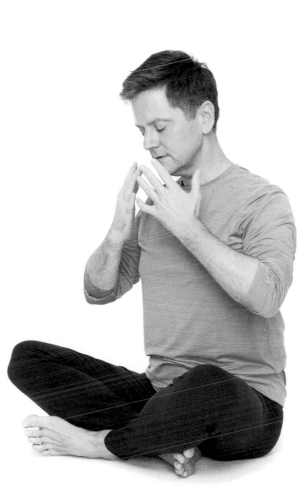

Transform Anxiety into Peace

———

Anxiety is a feeling of worry and unease over an event with an unclear outcome. This fear can be overwhelming. Whether in our personal lives or in politics, anxiety is on the rise. Our own well-being can be compromised because we're so busy trying to help others. So much feels out of our control.

When we don't manage our anxiety, it can have a negative impact on our lives. Unresolved anxiety affects our mental and physical health. Anxious thoughts create headaches, digestive issues, and muscle and joint pain.

Anxiety can be our teacher and show us that something needs to be addressed so we can find peace. Instead of focusing so much time and energy in the past or on fear of the future, anxiety can be a gentle reminder to feel safe in the present moment. It reminds us to breathe deeply to help quiet our mind and calm the nervous system. It helps us find balance by moving our attention from the mind into the body to explore sensations and to get grounded and connected.

This sequence is designed to help you manage your anxiety. Your mind may continue to race, but keep in mind that you are doing one pose at a time, one breath at a time. Your intention is to gently move from anxiety to peace.

JOURNALING PROMPT

I feel anxious because . . .

When I'm anxious, my body feels . . .

I'm worried about . . .

INTENTION

My intention is . . .

MOVING FORWARD

Put pen to paper: What's making you feel anxious and overwhelmed?

Take a break: Anxiety escalates when we're overthinking. When you feel anxious, deepen your breath and explore the sensations in your body. Take a break and walk away from the situation. Take time to focus on your body and relax your mind.

Repeat this affirmation: I relax and let all my feelings flow.

TRANSFORMATIVE FLOW

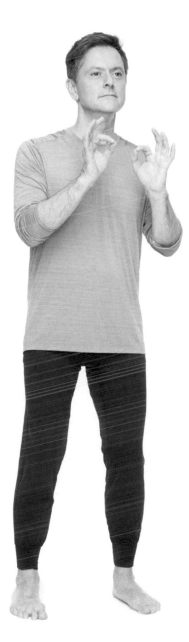

Transform Depression into Hope

When we are in loss, it's normal to feel numb and stuck. We can literally lose our way, feeling frustrated, exhausted, tired, and unsure how to move forward. We lose our passion, excitement, and hope and can become indifferent to life. We try to push through it, but most of the time, we feel exhausted and want to give up. In this state of unhappiness, it's hard to concentrate. We lack energy but find it hard to rest; our sleep patterns get disturbed. A hurricane of emotions may be whirling around, or we may feel bored and unmotivated.

Depression can be a teacher that encourages us to surrender. It can help put your feet back on the ground. It can be a place to nourish yourself and find renewal. By exploring depression, we can push through boundaries and release anger. Explore laughter exercises. Don't ignore, resist, or avoid what you're feeling. Lean into depression because these feelings can bring you intuitive wisdom. Tune in to what you're feeling and express it. Welcome them. Honor them. This too shall pass. Remind yourself that there is hope on the other side.

JOURNALING PROMPT

I feel hopeless and stuck because . . .

When I'm depressed, my body feels like . . .

I'm discouraged because . . .

INTENTION

My intention is . . .

MOVING FORWARD

Get outside: Take a walk and observe your surroundings. You are okay where you are right now. Even when you're feeling hopeless or worthless, remember that you matter.

Focus on connection: Find ways to develop connection and communication with yourself or someone you care about.

Repeat this affirmation: I am valued and worthy even when I'm not productive. I am a resilient silent warrior.

TRANSFORMATIVE FLOW

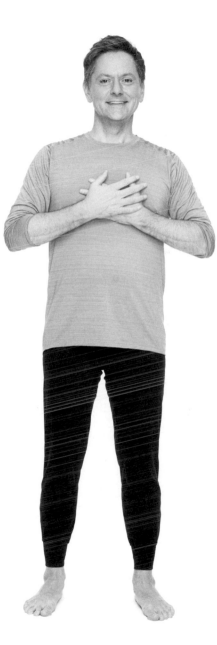

AFTERWORD

Finding Hope

After class, Rebecca, one of my students, said, "Ever since my husband died months ago, I haven't been able to feel happy or sad. I've just felt numb and depressed. This experience has given me hope."

"Is there a way you can bring more hope into your life?" I asked.

"I've felt so isolated and alone. Before Jim died, we talked a lot about getting a dog."

"Is it time to do that?"

She smiled and thanked me for the class. A few weeks later, she returned to class with a big smile on her face. "I did it," she said. "I got a dog. She's a sweet little light in my life. I call her Hope. I spend my days with her. Every day when I wake up, I see Hope. I've been walking and exercising with Hope. I'm meeting new people because of her. She's bringing more laughter into my life."

In Grief Yoga, I try to help people access hope like a light at the end of a tunnel. I'm secretly trying to guide people on a pathway to that hope. In a Grief Yoga class, it seems like it's about the postures, exercises, meditations, the dance or laughter, but it's actually about hope.

In Grief Yoga, I try to help people access hope like a light at the end of a tunnel.

254

My students often arrive at my class feeling hopeless, down, and sad. I invite them to believe that life is still worth living. I hold out hope for them, even if they can't find it for themselves. I guide them to believe that things will get better through work, connections, the divine, and perseverance.

Hope is ever-changing, and even in the most difficult times, it is there. We may progress from hoping we will have a long life with someone to hoping an illness isn't serious to hoping the person will have a peaceful death. Once they are gone, we can hope that we will be reunited someday and that we will live a life that honors the person who died.

Another client, Joseph, became bereaved when his daughter died. We spoke about how, ever since she was born, his hopes in life had mostly been wrapped up in her. She was smart and kind and wanted to grow up to be a veterinarian, to help animals. Joseph hoped that she would lead an incredible life, and his purpose was to help her achieve that incredible life. But she died at the age of eleven, and those hopes were gone.

New purpose can allow us to find new hope. Joseph worked to share his love for his daughter with others, and he did this by founding an animal shelter. In doing so, he chose to continue to live, to create something for his daughter and for others.

People talk often about planting a seed. But what's often forgotten is that planting a seed is a first step. There is so much work that has to follow in order for a seed to grow into a plant and then blossom. If your first step is planting a seed, what follows involves a series of choices. With Joseph, for example, he planted a seed when he *decided* he wanted to found an animal shelter to honor his daughter. But that decision alone wouldn't create an animal shelter overnight. He needed a location, staff, permits, licenses, and so much more. Sometimes in grief we only have the energy to plant a seed, but in time we can begin to nurture that seed so it grows.

Hope can and will help you evolve to create a good and happy life with your grief, but only if you do the work that hope requires. Know that your seed of hope has to continually be watered. Your life can bloom and blossom again, and you get to decide what it will become. What new life do you want to begin? Grief may end the life we used to live, but even as we close that chapter, we can turn the page and begin a new chapter. We get to write something entirely different. What will it be? Embrace a sense of mystery about hope. It will allow you to be curious. Just allowing the possibility of a good life can help you move forward. Ask yourself, *What can my life be now?*

Life is infinite. There is more purpose and love available to you. What can you let in?

Hope is our constant companion in this life. We always, always have it. But it's not unusual for people in grief to *feel* hopeless, though the hope is always there.

When people come into my class, I hold hope for each one of them. And I know that they have hope within themselves, too, because otherwise they wouldn't bother to come to class. Even if they can't see or feel their own hope, it is there, helping them seek the support they need. Hope is what brought you to this book. You have it, even if you don't always feel it. When I hear someone say, "I feel hopeless," I tell them, "I will hold your hope. I have hope for you, and I will hold it until you can feel it again."

This book is here, holding hope for you. You can find it here when you can't find it elsewhere. Hope lives within these pages, for you.

Contentment may still be some time away, but it is there for you, and it will come to you. Be gentle and compassionate with yourself so you can ease your suffering. Give yourself permission to be sad, to feel your feelings. Remember that this too shall pass—that permission is what will allow contentment to find its way to you.

As you practice Grief Yoga and seek contentment, reflect on these things:

- Accept what is.
- Let go what doesn't serve you.
- Focus on being present with your breath.
- Focus on something you're grateful for.
- Focus on what excites you and makes you and the people you love experience happiness.

This book is based on the cycle of compassionate transformation—but this is a cycle you can enter at any point. Do any exercise, in any order, and you will move forward and find your way to awareness, expression, connection, surrender, and evolution, over and over again, and each cycle will bring you closer to contentment.

If you allow yourself the space to feel whatever you're feeling, however painful, it will move through you. Be the observer of your breath and ask your body what wisdom it has to share. It always has something to tell you.

Just know, this too shall pass. The law of impermanence means that all things will pass.

Just know, this too shall pass. The law of impermanence means that all things will pass. This breath and moment shall pass. This life shall pass. You get to choose how to live today. How to love today. How to remember and honor those who have lived. What would they want for you today?

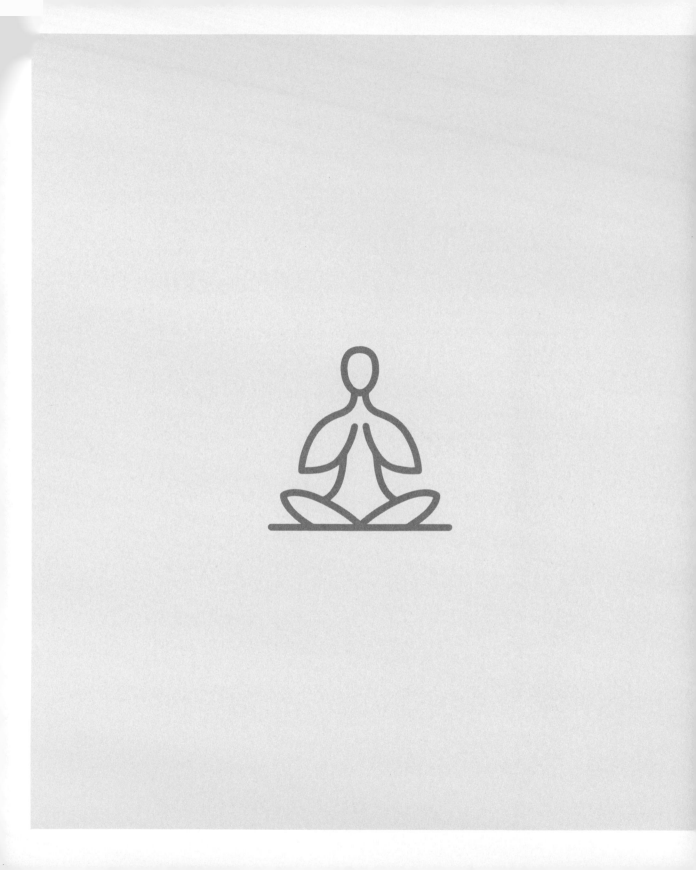

ACKNOWLEDGMENTS

I am humbled by the support I've received for many years to help bring this book to life. My agent, Leslie Meredith, is the angel who believed in me and helped me bring it to the world. At Chronicle Books, the guidance and care of my editor, Cara Bedick, has made this book into something even greater than I could have imagined. Her editing uplifts my work and helps others fully understand my intent. I couldn't have asked for a better editor on my first book. Jeff Campbell's copy-edit was the final touch to make my words become all they could be. Cecilia Santini offered wonderful suggestions and clarity. Cheyenne Ellis's pictures, creative eye, and caring heart have immensely enhanced this book with visuals. Thank you to Chronicle Prism, Mark Tauber, and Jenn Jensen for allowing the work to grow and expand in beautiful and meaningful ways, and for Pamela Geismar's artistic design to help bring beauty to this project.

Andrea Cagan has been my writing teacher and editor and inspired me to share, write, and speak from my authentic voice. Nikki Van De Car was an important light through the process. Martha Williams helped bring Grief Yoga to Kripalu Center for Yoga and Health and to 1440 Multiversity. Cheryl Fraenzl and Paula Wild have been there for me while I was teaching Grief Yoga at Esalen. Richard Dunkerley and Venetia David at Alternatives in the United Kingdom provided a sacred space where I could be of service to others. Hanna Nowicki at Tatra has been a strong guide in Australian teachings.

David Kessler has shown me so much love. His presence has made me a better man and allowed Grief Yoga to grow and expand in healing ways. Our love has made my life more meaningful. Nancy Levin's guidance was important when I wasn't sure if I could do this. Thank you to the teachers who have been my inspiration, like Bessel van der Kolk, Licia Sky, Bonnie MacBird, Ida Vernay, Gurmukh, and Seane Corn.

In my day-to-day work, Krista Richards, a true visionary, helped expand Grief Yoga into something greater online. Beth Segaloff is my rock and has helped make Grief Yoga a more meaningful experience.

My mom always offered me care and devotion. I will forever be her sweetheart man. My dad embodies a gentle giant and demonstrates what it is to be a humble servant. Thank you for loving me unconditionally my whole life. To my beloved sister, Ella, in heaven—the kindness and bond we shared will forever be in my heart. When we were growing up, you were always my best friend. I thank my brother, Kirk Denniston, for his artistic mind, laughter, and love. You are there whenever I need help. Colin Clayton's love, vulnerability, and laughter have made our family a better home.

John McCrite is my soul brother whose nuggets of wisdom, laughter, and forever friendship are invaluable to me. Greg Hoffman's friendship and love enrich me and make my life a more enjoyable ride. Juan Lopez's kindness and love are heartfelt offerings to my family. To my furry best friends, Angel and Lucy—thank you for teaching me how to be present and embody unconditional love.

To Lee Edmiston, Blake and Kyle Edmiston, and Travis Schubert for supporting my sister, Ella, and giving her so much love in her life. She lives on in you.

To all my students who have shown their love, vulnerability, and strength in my classes. To all the yoga teachers who have trained and become Grief Yoga teachers. You will always be a part of my tribe. To Megan Ducate, Terry Gloeggler, Amanda Larson-Mekler, and Abbe Andersen Starr for being my yoga angel teachers in the Grief Yoga online courses. To Patrick Allocca for his help in bringing the Grief Yoga videos to life. And to my dancing angel Jaquelin Levin-Zabare, for teaching me about the sacredness of life and reminding me to embrace more pleasure every day.

And to those in this book who have shared their love, loss, and ways to move forward—they will forever be my teachers.

ABOUT THE AUTHOR

Paul Denniston is the founder of Grief Yoga, which uses yoga, movement, breath, and sound to release pain and suffering and to connect to love.

Paul is certified in Hatha Yoga, Vinyasa Flow, Kundalini Yoga, Laughter Yoga, Restorative Yoga, and Let Your Yoga Dance. He also has taught movement at the Stella Adler Academy in Hollywood.

His intention with Grief Yoga is to combine many different forms of yoga in order to help heal grief. He has several online courses dealing with all kinds of loss and teaches this practice to counselors, psychologists, and health-care professionals on his training platform: Grief Movement Training. Paul certifies other yoga teachers in the Grief Yoga Teacher Training. He also teaches at Kripalu Center for Yoga and Health in Massachusetts, at Esalen, and at 1440 Multiversity.

Paul volunteered for years at one of the largest Los Angeles hospices, where he offered Heart Touch massage to the dying. He teaches Grief Yoga to bereavement groups; cancer support centers; groups whose loved ones died by suicide; Alzheimer's groups; groups for healing after a breakup, divorce, or betrayal; and addiction groups.

Paul has trained thousands of therapists, counselors, and health-care professionals in the United States, England, Ireland, Germany, and Australia. For more information, visit www.griefyoga.com.

INDEX